# COMMUNITY
# PHARMACY PRACTICE
# GUIDEBOOK

# COMMUNITY PHARMACY PRACTICE GUIDEBOOK

**Editors**

**Jessica Wooster, PharmD, BCACP**
Clinical Assistant Professor
Clinical Pharmacist, Ambulatory Care
Ben and Maytee Fisch College of Pharmacy
University of Texas
Tyler, Texas

**Frank S. Yu, PharmD**
Clinical Assistant Professor
Director, Advanced Pharmacy Practice Experiences
Ben and Maytee Fisch College of Pharmacy
University of Texas
Tyler, Texas

New York   Chicago   San Francisco   Athens   London   Madrid   Mexico City
Milan   New Delhi   Singapore   Sydney   Toronto

**Community Pharmacy Practice Guidebook**

1 2 3 4 5 6 7 8 9  LCR  27 26 25 24 23 22

ISBN 978-1-260-47026-0
MHID 1-260-47026-1

This book was set in Adobe Garamond by MPS Limited.
The editors were Michael Weitz and Peter J. Boyle.
The production supervisor was Rick Ruzycka.
Project management was provided by Poonam Bisht, MPS Limited.
The cover designer was W2 Design.

Cataloging-in-Publication data for this book is on file at the Library of Congress.

McGraw Hill books are available at special quantity discounts to use as premiums and sales promotions or for use in corporate training programs. To contact a representative, please visit the Contact Us pages at www.mhprofessional.com

# CONTENTS

# CONTRIBUTORS

**Jeremy Ashley, PharmD**
Clinical Assistant Professor
The University of Texas at Tyler, Ben and Maytee Fisch College of Pharmacy
Tyler, Texas
*Chapter 6*

Jeremy Ashley received his Doctor of Pharmacy from the Texas Tech University Health Sciences Center School of Pharmacy in Lubbock, Texas. He is a Clinical Assistant Professor at the University of Texas at Tyler Fisch College of Pharmacy. His clinical service involves consulting pharmacy in the long-term care (LTC) arena. As a consultant pharmacist, Dr. Ashley services several LTC facilities in the East Texas area, caring for over 700 patients. He ensures facilities remain up-to-date and compliant with CMS regulations, conducts clinical reviews as required by federal and state regulations, communicates early warning signs of potential problems to prescribers and nursing staff, and oversees and performs drug destruction for all discontinued and expired controlled and legend medications. Before academia and pharmacy consulting, Dr. Ashley practiced in the community pharmacy setting for 11 years and served in various roles, including pharmacy manager, pharmacy compliance liaison, and as a clinical pharmacist at the corporate level for two established retail grocery chains in Texas. Professional and research interests include Texas pharmacy law and regulatory affairs, geriatric pharmacy advancement, and pharmacist well-being and burnout prevention. He enjoys serving as faculty advisor for the TPA Academy of Student Pharmacists, as a member of the UT Tyler Admissions Committee, and as a member of the American Society of Consultant Pharmacists (ASCP). At the college, Dr. Ashley coordinates the Introduction to Pharmacy Practice Skills course and the Social-Behavioral Pharmacy and Practice Management course and offers an APPE Consultant Pharmacy elective that focuses on the geriatric population.

**Rachel E. Barenie, PharmD, JD, MPH**
Assistant Professor, Department of Clinical Pharmacy and Translational Science
Assistant Director, Office of Continuing Professional Development
The University of Tennessee Health Science Center, College of Pharmacy
Memphis, Tennessee
*Chapter 5*

Rachel E. Barenie is a pharmacist and attorney by training. She also completed a Postdoctoral Fellowship in Pharmaceutical Policy at Harvard Medical School and Brigham and Women's Hospital in the Program on Regulation, Therapeutics, and Law ("PORTAL") from 2018–2020. During that time, she also began serving as a clinical consultant to Alosa Health, a not-for-profit academic detailing organization, for opioid use disorder-related content, a role that she continues to serve in. After her fellowship, she joined faculty at the University of Tennessee Health Science Center in July 2020. Currently, she is an Assistant Professor in the UTHSC College of Pharmacy and Assistant Director of the Office of Continuing Professional Development in the college.

**Vanessa Brown, PharmD**
Pharmacy Operations Specialist
McKesson HealthMart
Las Colinas, Texas
*Chapter 7*

Vanessa Brown graduated from the University of Texas College of Pharmacy in 2006 but has been working in a pharmacy since 1999. She worked for a large chain as a pharmacy manager for almost 10 years until she turned her focus to the independent world. From there, she started a consulting company that helped independent pharmacies with their compliance programs as well as helping them discover diverse revenue streams. Today she is the Pharmacy Operations Specialist for Health Mart, an independent pharmacy franchise from McKesson that serves over 5000 independent pharmacies. She helps to ensure that programs, products, and resources available from Health Mart effectively support its customers.

**Jay Bueche, RPh**
Director of Pharmacy—Managed Care
H-E-B
San Antonio, Texas
*Chapter 9*

Jay Bueche received his Bachelor of Pharmacy from the University of Texas in Austin in 1995. After working in a variety of store locations and roles, including pharmacy manager, he joined the H-E-B Pharmacy corporate management team in 2004. Jay's experience has included quality improvement, regulatory compliance and, since 2010, third party and managed care. In his current role, Jay leads a team responsible for payer relations, contracting, store support (e.g., audits, claim troubleshooting) and pricing. Additionally, Jay is responsible for monitoring and advocating for changes in payment policy at the Federal and State level. He has served as a preceptor for several Texas Colleges of Pharmacy spreading his passion for advocacy and involvement. Jay has served as president of the Texas Federation of Drug Stores, vice president of the Texas Pharmacy Association and on committees and boards for several other associations and organizations.

**Raj Chhadua, PharmD, RPh**
Managing Partner
Renue Apothecary GP
Frisco, Texas
*Chapter 2*

Raj Chhadua, PharmD, currently serves as the managing partner for Renue Apothecary GP that owns and manages 10 independent pharmacies in the state of Texas and Iowa. In addition to his work responsibilities, he previously served as the Texas Pharmacy Association President to continue to advocate and protect the profession of pharmacy. Dr. Chhadua previously worked for the Walgreen Company for 18 years serving in his last role as the Health Care Supervisor for the Dallas Fort Worth region until April 2016. In 2007, as the Walgreens immunization leader for North, Central, and West Texas, he was instrumental in transforming each of Walgreens' 296 stores in these areas into Immunization Centers of Excellence and seamlessly executed a program to provide immunization training and certification to the 675 pharmacists working in these stores. Dr. Chhadua earned a Doctorate in Pharmacy from Texas Tech University Health Science Center in 2002.

**Rannon Ching, PharmD**
Pharmacist in Charge
Tarrytown Pharmacy
Austin, Texas
*Chapter 9*

Rannon is the Pharmacist in Charge at Tarrytown Pharmacy, an independent pharmacy that has been serving the community of Austin Texas since 1941. He was born in Honolulu Hawaii, living there until his family moved to Lake Travis in Austin, Texas in 2000. Rannon completed his undergraduate prerequisites and his Doctor of Pharmacy at the University of Texas at Austin in 2014. He manages and operates Tarrytown Pharmacy, an Austin-based independent pharmacy, and their numerous advanced clinical services; including their PGY-1 community pharmacy residency, immunization and point-of-care testing program, third and fourth year IPPE and APPE UT College of Pharmacy students, and healthcare facility relations. The Texas Pharmacy Association awarded him with the 2019 Excellence in Innovation award, which recognizes an individual who has demonstrated innovative pharmacy practice resulting in improved patient care and/or advancement of the profession of pharmacy. Rannon was also honored with the 2019 Distinguished Young Alumnus Award from the UT Austin College of Pharmacy Alumni Association. He currently serves as the Speaker for the Texas Pharmacy Association's House of Delegates. He works closely with the University of Texas at Austin College of Pharmacy, and is involved with teaching third- and fourth-year pharmacy students, developing research projects, and is a member of the college's Experiential and Admissions committee. In addition, he equips and encourages his pharmacy team to pursue new and innovative advanced clinical services for the pharmacy.

**Mark Comfort, PharmD**
Pharmacy Manager
H-E-B Grocery
Austin, Texas
*Chapter 4*

Dr. Mark Comfort received his Doctor of Pharmacy from the University of Texas at Austin, College of Pharmacy in 2003. He has worked as a pharmacy manager for H-E-B Grocery for over 15 years. During this time he has managed 5 different pharmacy locations for H-E-B. Each of these locations varied in customer demographics, pharmacy layout, script volume, and staff size. For over 10 years, Mark managed one of the busiest community pharmacies in Texas. He also serves as Preceptor-Faculty for the University of Texas College of Pharmacy and precepts students in all years of pharmacy school. In addition, Mark has served as a Preceptor for the H-E-B/UT PGY1 Community-based Pharmacy Residency Program. Mark is very active in professional organizations and has served on the boards of the Capital Area Pharmacy Association (Austin, TX) and the Texas Pharmacy Association. He has served as Director, Secretary, and President of the Capital Area Pharmacy Association, and has also served as Vice-President and President of the Texas Pharmacy Association. Mark is the 2018–2019 recipient of the Pharmacy Leadership Award presented by the National Community Pharmacists Association (NCPA).

**James Cong, PharmD**
Director of Clinical Affairs
Tarrytown Pharmacy
Austin, Texas
*Chapter 10*

Dr. Cong is the Director of Clinical Affairs at Tarrytown Pharmacy in Austin, Texas. In this role, he has worked to expand the outpatient clinical services to become a primary practice model. James has expanded Tarrytown Pharmacy's COVID-19 testing operations to 5 sites across Austin and worked to execute a Statewide vaccination effort for patients with intellectual or developmental disorders. He is passionate about doing whatever it takes to fill in the gaps of care that can occur along the way in the healthcare process.

**Tyler Dinkelaker, PharmD, JD, MBA**
Compliance Manager
Lemonaid Pharmacy
St. Louis, Missouri
*Chapter 5*

Tyler Dinkelaker is a pharmacist and compliance manager for a nationally licensed telemedicine provider. He grew up working in his parent's pharmacy, holding just about every job possible from clerk to pharmacist and compounding manager upon graduation from the St. Louis College of Pharmacy (now University of Health Sciences in St. Louis.) Thereafter, he attended Saint Louis University Law School and University of Missouri, St. Louis, earning both his JD and MBA. Currently, he focuses his work on helping companies define and establish robust compliance programs while enabling their team leaders to innovate within the United States' federal and state level laws and regulations. He also spends time mentoring local college and graduate students and providing legal review sessions for pharmacy graduates in the St. Louis Area.

**Will Douglas, PharmD**
Owner
Crimson Care Pharmacy Group
Dallas, Texas
*Chapter 7*

Will Douglas is a self-made multi-site pharmacy owner who grew up in a small town in Southern Oklahoma. Will paid his way through the University of Oklahoma College of Pharmacy before moving to Dallas to begin his career. Through hard work and long hours, Will purchased several small pharmacies and currently manages his own business, Crimson Care Pharmacy Group. Named one of Dallas County's "40 under 40" in 2019, Crimson Care was founded to ensure independently owned community pharmacies continue to survive and thrive in a changing healthcare environment that includes large-pharmacy chain expansion, buyouts, and customer demand for the latest technology.

**Jeffrey Hamper, PharmD, BCACP**
Manager, Pharmacy Experiential, Internship, and Residency Programs
Albertsons Companies
Boise, Idaho
*Chapter 1*

Jeffrey Hamper started his career in community pharmacy before even applying to pharmacy school. Over the summers during college, he worked as a part-time stock clerk at a local supermarket. He would often have patients ask him questions that he referred to the pharmacist. He began overhearing the knowledgeable advice and recommendations from the pharmacist that customers would get right there in the aisles. After a couple of summers, Dr. Hamper decided to take the leap and apply for a pharmacy technician position with the same company and soon after applied to pharmacy school. During his first year of pharmacy school, he vividly remembers a lecture in one of his introductory courses about the roles and practice areas in pharmacy. It was about the relatively new field of Medication Therapy Management (MTM), and he knew right away that was what he thought all community pharmacists should do. Jeff completed a couple of summer internships in the community pharmacy setting, took some advanced community APPE rotations, and completed a PGY1 Community-based Pharmacy Residency Program which was one of the most formative experiences of his career so far. After residency, he managed a pharmacy for a couple of years while also serving as a community-based clinical pharmacist. He kept asking for more and more opportunities and responsibilities until he ultimately applied for his current role leading the community-based residency programs, internships, and experiential programs for his organization nationwide.

**Donald C. Hohmeier, CPA-Retired**
Cleveland, Ohio
*Chapter 8*

Donald C. Hohmeier practiced for 36 years before his retirement in 2016. Following his graduation with a BBA in Accounting from Cleveland State University in Cleveland OH, he began his career with a regional CPA firm where he counseled clients in a diverse range of industries from Manufacturing to Real Estate Development to Professional Services. Following his early career in public accounting and then as controller to a large real estate development organization, he served as chief financial officer to companies in Public Relations and Media where he also held positions on the Board of Directors and Executive Committee. He has been a guest lecturer at Kent State University and has presented various internal training programs on "The Business of Our Business."

**Kenneth C. Hohmeier, PharmD**
Associate Professor
University of Tennessee Health Science Center, College of Pharmacy
Nashville, Tennessee
*Chapters 2 and 8*

Kenneth C. Hohmeier, PharmD, is an Associate Professor and Director of Community Affairs in the Department of Clinical Pharmacy and Translational Science at the University of Tennessee Health Science Center. Dr. Hohmeier has an extensive background in pharmacy practice and practice-based and implementation science research, including post-graduate residency training in community pharmacy, credentials in lean six sigma, implementation science, the Innovator's DNA, and change leadership. He has successfully established and provided clinical pharmacist services within several community pharmacy settings in a wide variety of rural, suburban, and urban locations. His background also includes extensive leadership experience both in practice and within professional organizations, with past and current positions held at local, regional, and national levels including the American Pharmacists Association, Ohio Pharmacists Association, and Tennessee Public Health Association. His specific areas of research focus are in clinical service implementation in community pharmacy settings, MTM, and innovative clinical pharmacy practice models. He has served as Primary Investigator (PI) or Co-PI on over 15 grant-funded projects advancing the role of the community pharmacist to increase patient care activities, such as vaccinations, MTM, and other clinical services. He is the Residency Program Director for the UTHSC Community-based Pharmacy Residency Program, teaches in several courses throughout the UTHSC PharmD curriculum, and directs the Healthcare Leadership, Innovation, and Management course.

**Michelle Jeon, PharmD, BCACP**
Assistant Professor of Pharmacy Practice
St. Louis College of Pharmacy at UHSP
Shared Community Practice Faculty
Walgreens Pharmacy
St. Louis, Missouri
*Chapter 3*

Michelle Jeon received her Bachelor in Science and Doctor of Pharmacy from Philadelphia College of Pharmacy at University of the Sciences. She then decided to pursue community pharmacy and academia through the completion of a PGY1 Community Pharmacy Residency and subsequent faculty appointment at St. Louis College of Pharmacy at UHSP. She currently serves as an assistant professor of pharmacy practice, as well as residency program director for the PGY1 Walgreens/St. Louis College of Pharmacy at UHSP Community-Based Pharmacy Residency Program. Michelle's current practice site is at Walgreens Pharmacy, where she provides MTM services, immunization/travel health consultations, and HIV medication management.

**Jennifer Konieczny, PharmD**
Pharmacy Manager
Brookshire Grocery Company
Tyler, Texas
*Chapter 3*

Jennifer Konieczny received her Doctor of Pharmacy from the University of Colorado where she worked in community pharmacy for independent and chain pharmacies. As a Pharmacy Manager at CVS Pharmacy, she trained as a Pharmacy Supervisor Emerging Leader candidate, expanding her managerial and leadership skills. Jennifer moved to Brookshire's Grocery Company, where she has been for the past 4 years, and was the recipient of the Pharmacy Manager of the Year award in 2019.

**Nathan D. Pope, PharmD, BCACP, FACA**
Clinical Associate Professor
The University of Texas at Austin, College of Pharmacy
Austin, Texas
*Chapter 4*

Dr. Nathan Pope is Clinical Associate Professor and Assistant Division Head of Pharmacy Practice at The University of Texas at Austin College of Pharmacy. He received his B.S. and Pharm.D. from the Ernest Mario School of Pharmacy at Rutgers: The State University of New Jersey. Afterwards, he completed a Postgraduate (PGY1) Community Pharmacy-based Residency with Walgreens at the University of Houston College of Pharmacy. After residency, he worked in various community pharmacy-based settings ranging from a large national chain, a small regional chain, and independent pharmacy. Nathan is highly active in professional organizations having served on the boards of the Capital Area Pharmacy Association (Austin, TX), Texas Pharmacy Association, and the American College of Apothecaries. In addition, he has served as President of the Capital Area Pharmacy Association. Nathan is the Residency Program Director for the H-E-B/UT PGY1 Community-based Pharmacy Residency Program, Co-Director of the Lester Entrepreneurial Scholars Program, and Co-Director of the Teaching and Leadership Fellows Program at the College of Pharmacy. He is a recipient of the Bowl of Hygeia Award and has also been honored as Professor of the Semester by The University of Texas at Austin's Senate of College Councils.

**Chelsea P. Renfro, PharmD**
Assistant Professor
The University of Tennessee Health Science Center College of Pharmacy
Memphis, Tennessee
*Chapter 10*

Dr. Renfro is an Assistant Professor in the Department of Clinical Pharmacy and Translational Science at the University of Tennessee Health Science Center College of Pharmacy. Her academic interests focus on using simulation-based education to teach community pharmacy practice and self-care. Her primary research focuses on implementation of clinical pharmacy services in the community pharmacy setting. Through her research, she hopes to change the way community pharmacy is portrayed and delivered while influencing reimbursements strategies affecting health policy.

**Megan Rhyne, PharmD**
Pharmacy Manager
Brookshire Grocery Company
Tyler, Texas
*Chapter 3*

Megan Rhyne began her career in pharmacy when she was just 18 years old as a pharmacy clerk. She went on to get her national certification and worked as a technician for 4 years during undergrad where she received her Bachelor of Science from the University of Texas at Tyler. From there, she attended Texas A&M College of Pharmacy. Upon graduation, she worked as a staff pharmacist for a year before being promoted to pharmacy manager. Megan has now been a pharmacy manager for 7 years.

**Carol A. Schwab, JD, LLM**
Professor, College of Graduate Health Sciences
Professor, College of Pharmacy
University of Tennessee Health Science Center
Memphis, Tennessee
*Chapter 5*

Carol A. Schwab is an attorney by training, but she has been an educator for more than 30 years. After clerking for a federal judge and practicing law during the first 10 years of her career, she joined the faculty at NC State University, where for nearly 16 years, she taught legal seminars to the general public, focusing on estate planning, advance directives, and other end-of-life issues. At NCSU, she achieved the rank of tenured full professor. She received a number of awards, including a national award, for her programming efforts on aging. While in North Carolina, she was active in the North Carolina Bar Association, serving as editor for two different bar publications and serving as Chair for the Elder Law Section. She joined the faculty at the Medical College of Georgia in 2004 as a full professor and assistant dean and developed and implemented a curriculum for medical students on the Legal Issues of Medicine. She joined the faculty at the University of Tennessee Health Science Center in 2007 as a full professor and as the Director of Medical/Legal Issues, where she developed and implemented a similar curriculum for the UTHSC College of Medicine. From 2009 through 2020, she taught the required pharmacy law course in the UTHSC College of Pharmacy. Currently, she is a Full Professor in the UTHSC College of Graduate Health Sciences and teaches legal issues in health law to medical students and physician assistant students.

**Mark Sullivan, BPharm**
Pharmacy Operation Manager
Brookshire Grocery Company
Tyler, Texas
*Chapter 6*

Mark Sullivan received his Bachelor's in Pharmacy from the University of Mississippi School of Pharmacy in Oxford, Mississippi. He is the Pharmacy Operation Manager for Brookshire Grocery Company and a member of the Brookshires Corporate Development Team. His current position involves oversight of a 45 000-square foot automated central fill pharmacy housing 45 employees and serving 120 BGC retail pharmacies. In addition, Mr. Sullivan is responsible for the company's 340B program, third-party contract management, pricing and reimbursement integrity, Specialty Pharmacy compliance and DIR evaluation and strategy development. Before taking his current position with Brookshires, Mr. Sullivan served as the Director of Pharmacy for Medicine Chest Pharmacies, a regional retail and long-term care pharmacy provider. Prior to that, Mr. Sullivan was the owner/operator of Good's Pharmacies, Med-Care Long Term Care Pharmacy and Good's Home Infusion Pharmacy all located in Tyler, Texas. Professional and research interests include DIR evaluation and mitigation strategy, macroeconomic and political implication on pharmacy and collaborative practice development.

**Lance Thompson, PharmD**
Director of Education
Liberty Pharmacy Software
Southlake, Texas
*Chapter 7*

Lance Thompson cut his teeth behind the counter of independent pharmacies for 9 years before he began working for Liberty Pharmacy Software. As Liberty's Director of Education, he educates thousands of pharmacists and technicians on new technology and programs being developed. He regularly converses with pharmacy technology companies to understand the latest developments within the field. Lance also serves as a compounding pharmacist for clinical trials, where he works with emerging therapies for vision loss.

**Roxane L. Took, PharmD, BCACP**
Assistant Professor of Pharmacy Practice
St. Louis College of Pharmacy at University of Health Sciences and Pharmacy in St. Louis
St. Louis, Missouri
Clinical Pharmacist
Gateway Apothecary
St. Louis, Missouri
*Chapter 11*

Dr. Roxane Took received her Doctorate of Pharmacy from Southern Illinois University of Edwardsville in Edwardsville, Illinois and is a Board Certified Ambulatory Care Pharmacist. She is an Assistant Professor at St. Louis College of Pharmacy. Her practice site is at Gateway Apothecary, an independent pharmacy in St. Louis. As a clinical pharmacist, she completes MTM services for a little over 1000 patients at both Gateway Apothecary and Beverly Hills Pharmacy. The pharmacy also services a local physician's office through a clinical services agreement to provide annual wellness visits, chronic care management, remote physiologic management and behavioral health interventions. In 2014, Dr. Took completed a community-based PGY1 residency with Balls Food Stores in Kansas City where she initiated a transitions of care program for employees and dependents of Balls Food Stores. She also provided disease state management for employees and dependents with diabetes, hypertension, dyslipidemia, and acute coronary syndromes (i.e. myocardial infarction). She has experience in various community pharmacy settings (chain, grocery store, and independent) and with a variety of clinical services. She enjoys serving as a faculty advisor for the student chapter of Missouri Pharmacy Association, a member-at-large on the Missouri Pharmacy Association Board of Directors, co-chair for the American Pharmacists Association Transitions of Care Communication Committee, and member of various pharmacy organizations.

**Angelina Tucker, PharmD, BCGP**
Managing Network Facilitator
CPESN-Texas
Clinical Pharmacist
Best Value Pharmacies, Inc.
Fort Worth, Texas
*Chapter 11*

Dr. Angelina Tucker earned her Bachelor of Pharmacy from the University of the West Indies in Trinidad and Tobago and her Doctor of Pharmacy from the University of Florida in Gainesville Florida and is a Board Certified Geriatric Pharmacist. She is the clinical director for a chain of 13 independent pharmacies where she manages the chain's MTM services, diabetes self-management education (DSME) classes and community engagement/networking. Dr. Tucker serves as a preceptor for students in an MTM and a geriatric ambulatory APPE rotation. She is also the Managing Network Facilitator of Community Pharmacy Enhanced Services Network (CPESN) Texas, her role includes expanding the network and driving the market for value-based payment models in Texas and mentoring pharmacies through the DSME accreditation process. Dr. Tucker has been a public educator for the past 25 years, empowering senior citizens in the community, independent and assisted living facilities to reclaim their medical autonomy to promote healthy aging in place. In her prior role as pharmacy director at a private hospital, Dr. Tucker provided care services in cardiology and oncologic clinics. Her experience as pharmacy manager at a chain pharmacy developed her community networking skills to increase sales, engagement and education. Dr. Tucker is a member of and a speaker at the ASCP.

**Benjamin Y. Urick, PharmD**
Assistant Professor
University of North Carolina, Eshelman School of Pharmacy
Chapel Hill, North Carolina
*Chapter 10*

Dr. Urick is an Assistant Professor in the Center for Medication Optimization at the UNC Eshelman School of Pharmacy. His academic interests lie at the intersection of pharmacy practice, healthcare, and health policy. His primary research focuses on the role of community pharmacists in the evolving healthcare system and the use of secondary data to measure healthcare quality and spending. His current research includes evaluation of pharmacy services interventions, scientific reliability of provider-level quality measures, and factors which influence medication-related healthcare quality.

**Robert Willis, PharmD, BCACP**
Residency Program Director/Corporate Pharmacy Trainer
Albertsons Companies
Centennial, Connecticut
*Chapter 1*

Robert Willis embarked on his pharmacy career as a pharmacy clerk and quickly found his passion for community pharmacy. After 6 months of working in the pharmacy, he obtained his pharmacy technician certification and changed his college major from pre-medicine to pre-pharmacy. During pharmacy school, he obtained an internship at a supermarket community pharmacy. During his internship he was exposed to novel community pharmacy practice and this innovation ignited his passion for advancing community pharmacy practice. After Robert graduated from pharmacy school, he managed a local supermarket pharmacy and began to help advance practice by implementing numerous clinical services. He was an early adopter of MTM, Travel Health Services and Point-of-Care testing. He also helped implement diabetes management, medication administration, and smoking cessation services and training and even had the opportunity to refine the pharmacist's clinical role at a drug and alcohol recovery center. In 2014, Robert began his journey as a Community-based Residency Program Director (RPD). His role as an RPD was the next step in helping advance community pharmacy practice. Currently, Robert is an RPD and a Corporate Pharmacy Trainer. Once again, he has found himself in a dual role that allows him to help advance the profession.

# PREFACE

Greetings, pharmacy students, preceptors, and faculty. This textbook, or more appropriately, guidebook, was created to fill an unmet need in the Doctor of Pharmacy curricula. While a significant portion of didactic curricula relevant to community pharmacy includes topics such as communication, pharmacotherapy, self-care, and other patient care skills, other non-clinical facets of community pharmacy practice may be missing. Based on feedback from pharmacists and faculty nationwide, community pharmacy topics such as human resource management, workflow optimization, implementing value-based clinical services, and other practice-based topics are typically covered in either electives or experiential education, if at all.

The goal of our guidebook is to introduce learners to content relevant to community pharmacy practice in the didactic setting. While this is not meant to replace any of the existing textbooks currently in use, we hope that it will serve in a standalone or complementary capacity in the curriculum. This text is intended for pharmacy students prior to embarking on their community pharmacy Introductory Pharmacy Practice Experiences (IPPE), giving them a practical understanding of different responsibilities of the community pharmacist. This text can also be used by community pharmacy preceptors on either IPPE or Advanced Pharmacy Practice Experiences (APPE) to serve as a foundation for topic discussions and other learning activities.

Students and community pharmacy preceptors frequently comment that what is taught in the classroom does not mirror what occurs in real life. For this reason, each chapter of this guidebook intentionally includes authors who are full-time community pharmacists, pharmacy practice faculty, and experts in the content area (e.g. CPA and attorneys). This was done to provide learners with practical, real-life content relevant to what they need to know in community pharmacy practice, in a format that can be used in the classroom or experiential setting. We believe that you will find this guidebook relevant, concise, and practical.

# 1.

# COMMUNITY PHARMACY PRACTICE AND PHARMACY DESIGN MODELS

*Jeffrey Hamper, PharmD, BCACP, and Robert Willis, PharmD, BCACP*

---

## ■ LEARNING OBJECTIVES

1. List the types of community pharmacies and pharmacy personnel roles.
2. Identify the services, both operational and patient care, offered at a community pharmacy.
3. Describe the advancement of the community pharmacist's role.
4. Discuss the factors that are considered when designing a community pharmacy.
5. Describe examples of innovative community-based pharmacy practice models.

## ■ SETTING THE SCENE

Community pharmacy practice is continuously evolving, and for us to know where the profession is going, it is important to know where we have been. Throughout history, as long as there was disease, illness, or injury to treat, roles like that of the community pharmacist have existed in forms such as medicine men, shamans, and healers.[1] The concept of the distinct pharmacist role arose in medieval Islamic culture. By the mid-13th century, German emperor Frederick II issued his edict for the profession of pharmacy that established pharmacy as an independent branch of governmentally supervised health service. This was created by separating the pharmaceutical profession from the medical profession, requiring official supervision of pharmaceutical practice, and an obligation by oath to prepare drugs reliably in a uniform, suitable quality.[2]

In colonial America and the early Republic, apothecary shop practice began to evolve and by the 18th through the mid-19th centuries, pharmacists were manufacturing ingredients and preparations in their shops.[1,3] Between the 1820s and the 1940s, pharmacists served as compounders of prescriptions, and the classic American drugstore arose. From the 1930s to the mid-1960s, more effective drugs were developed and trends of prescribing individual drugs rather than compounded medications increased, which further resulted in the era of the "count and pour" dispenser and development of the chain drug industry.[1,3] Through the mid-1960s to 1990, the profession of pharmacy began to diversify as the role of hospital pharmacy and clinical pharmacy emerged.[1,3] With the passage of the Omnibus Budget Reconciliation Act of 1990, pharmacists were brought into the pharmaceutical care era, as federal law now set a practice standard and a set of responsibilities for pharmacists. Finally, with the passage of the Medicare Modernization Act of 2003, the concept of medication therapy management (MTM) was born. As this cognitive service was now independent of medication products, this led us to the era of MTM and provider status.[1,3]

While this history was extremely brief and certainly not all-inclusive, this gives us a glimpse into the prospective future role of the community pharmacist, which may not always include dispensing medications. The vision of the American Pharmacists Association (APHA) adopted by their Board of Trustees adopted in 2017 was "The American Pharmacists Association inspires, innovates, and creates opportunities for members and pharmacists worldwide to optimize medication use and health for all..."[4] In 2015, the Joint Commission of Pharmacy Practitioners (JCPP), a group of national pharmacy organizations that was established in 1977, issued their "Vision of Pharmacy Practice" that pharmacists will provide services within community-based practices, institutions, clinics, patients' homes, or other settings, and will coordinate, collaborate, and communicate among themselves and with other members of the healthcare team.[5] It is clear, based on the evolution of community pharmacy practice and the vision of major pharmacy organizations, that the profession of pharmacy will continue to evolve from primarily a dispensing role to one focused on direct patient care as part of the greater healthcare team. The way pharmacy is practiced and the design of pharmacies themselves must continue to evolve to assist us in this professional transformation.

There are numerous community pharmacies located throughout the United States, and many Doctor of Pharmacy programs require student pharmacists to complete various Introductory Pharmacy Practice Experiences (IPPE) and Advanced Pharmacy Practice Experiences (APPE) within the community pharmacy setting. This chapter will provide insight into the design of community pharmacies and what the student pharmacist may expect to see the first time that they step into a community pharmacy.

# COMMUNITY PHARMACY PRACTICE

## Types of Community Pharmacies and Organizational Structure

Pharmacists continue to rank highly as one of the most trusted professions, according to the 2019 Gallup's Honest and Ethics survey.[6] In addition, pharmacists are one of the most easily accessible healthcare professionals and 90% of Americans live within 5 miles of a community pharmacy.[7] Community pharmacies play a pivotal role within the communities that they serve. Community pharmacies offer numerous services including traditional core operations and patient care services, where allowed by state law. See Figure 1-1.

There are many types of community pharmacies including independently owned pharmacies and chain pharmacies.[8] See Figure 1-2. The type of community pharmacy and the state's pharmacy practice act will impact the type of services offered within the pharmacy. Community pharmacies are located throughout the country in remote, rural locations, and metropolitan areas. The geographical location of community pharmacies may also impact the types of services that the pharmacy offers.

Each community pharmacy will have its own unique organizational chart that shows the relationship among various roles and positions within the pharmacy department. An independent pharmacy's organizational chart may include the pharmacy owner,

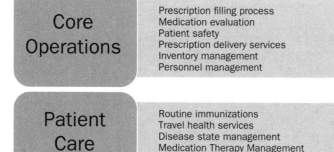

**Core Operations**
Prescription filling process
Medication evaluation
Patient safety
Prescription delivery services
Inventory management
Personnel management

**Patient Care Services**
Routine immunizations
Travel health services
Disease state management
Medication Therapy Management
Medication administration
Pharmacist prescribing

**Figure 1-1.** Community pharmacy example operations and services.

**Large Retail Pharmacy**
CVS
Rite-Aid
Walgreens

**Mass Merchandiser**
Costco
Walmart

**Supermarket-Based Pharmacy**
Albertsons Companies
Kroger
Publix

**Figure 1-2.** Types of chain pharmacies with examples.

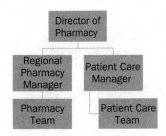

**Figure 1-3.** Example chain organizational chart, upper management.

pharmacy manager, and pharmacy staff. Chain community pharmacies' organizational charts are often more robust due to multiple locations and corporate pharmacy structure. See Figures 1-3 and 1-4 for examples of chain organizational charts.

The various roles and responsibilities within a chain community pharmacy organization include:

*Director of Pharmacy*: Oversees the business operations and patient care services offered in a geographic region, multiple pharmacy locations, and, possibly, in a multi-state.

*Patient Care Manager*: Manages the patient care services offered in a geographic region, multiple pharmacy locations, and, possibly, in a multi-state.

*Patient Care Team*: Provides remote and on-site patient care services.

*Regional Pharmacy Manager*: Manages the business operations of multiple pharmacy locations.

*Pharmacy Manager/Pharmacist in Charge* (PIC): Manages business operations and patient care services at one pharmacy location.

*Staff Pharmacist*: Supports the Pharmacy Manager by helping with business operations and patient care services. Operates as PIC when the Pharmacy Manager is not present.

*Pharmacy Resident (Pharmacist)*: Supports business operations and offers patient care services, while completing a structured post-graduate training program.

*Pharmacy Intern*: Aids in business operations and pharmacy services, while completing pharmacy school. Completes pharmacist-type functions, under the supervision of the pharmacist. This can be either as

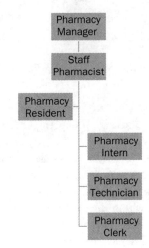

**Figure 1-4.** Example chain organizational chart, pharmacy team.

a paid employee of the pharmacy or as a student as part of their IPPE or APPE experience.

*Pharmacy Technician*: Supports the pharmacy team with business operations and patient care services.

*Pharmacy Clerk*: Supports the pharmacy team with business operations and patient care services. Role and tasks are heavily restricted by state regulations.

### Advancing the Community Pharmacists' Role

Pharmacy priorities will vary depending on the type of pharmacy, company mission and goals, and pharmacy metrics. Prescription volume may play a role in overall pharmacy priorities. In general, supermarket pharmacies operate at a lower prescription volume as compared to a large retail pharmacy. For example, a supermarket pharmacy may only dispense 500 prescriptions in a given week as compared to a large retail pharmacy which may dispense up to several thousand prescriptions per week. Due to a lower prescription volume, some pharmacies may have more time to offer advanced patient care services such as immunizations, medication administration, and/or pharmacist prescribing services. Pharmacies may also be partnered with various types of clinics (e.g., urgent care clinic) to help meet the needs of their community. Some states have expanded the pharmacy technician role to aid the pharmacist in optimizing patient care. The technicians expanded role may include transcribing new prescriptions over the phone, tech-check-tech (final verification) of medication verification, administering immunizations, and/or technician prescribing (e.g., naloxone).

Community-based pharmacist practitioner (CPP) is a term that was coined to describe a pharmacist who provides patient care to the communities in any community-based setting.[9] Community-based pharmacies employ about 58% of pharmacists. *The Journal of the American Pharmacist Association* (JAPhA) provided commentary on CPPs and suggested four tenets of CPPs:

- Provides direct patient care to meet the healthcare needs of patients in the communities they serve
- Creates, advances, and influences team-based care to the benefit of patients they serve
- Strives to enhance management of community-based practice settings, their local communities, and within the profession of pharmacy
- Serves as a leader within community-based pharmacy settings, their local communities, and within the profession of pharmacy[10]

It is vital for community pharmacists to continue to elevate their pharmacy practice in their role as a CPP. To help structure the patient care experience, CPPs should use the JCPP—Pharmacists' Patient Care Process (PPCP) to provide comprehensive care to all patients.

The vision for pharmacists' practice by the JCPP is "Patients achieve optimal health and medication outcomes with pharmacists as essential and accountable providers within patient-centered, team-based healthcare." In 2014, JCPP released a follow-up document to this vision that listed their recommended pharmacist responsibilities. It stated that as members of the patient-centered healthcare team, pharmacists will be accountable for health, medication-related, and patient and population-specific needs by assuming responsibility for:

- Rational, evidence-based use of medications
- Facilitating achievement of patients' health and medication-related goals

- Promotion of wellness, health improvement, and disease prevention
- Design and oversight of safe, accurate, and timely medication distribution systems
- Provision of high-quality, compassionate, cost-effective care[5]

In 2014, the JCPP also released the PPCP which is now widely taught in PharmD curricula and pharmacy residency programs across the country.[11] In the PPCP, pharmacists use a patient-centered approach to optimize patient health and medication outcomes by collaborating with other providers on the healthcare team. See Figure 1-5 for a visual representation of this process. Using principles of evidence-based practice, pharmacists: collect and assess patient information, develop and implement individualized care plans in collaboration with other healthcare professionals and the patient, monitor and evaluate the effectiveness of the care plans, and modify the plan in collaboration with the healthcare team and patient as needed. The JCPP PPCP should be implemented by all pharmacists, regardless of their primary practice setting or patient care service, to ensure a consistent process in the delivery of patient care.[11]

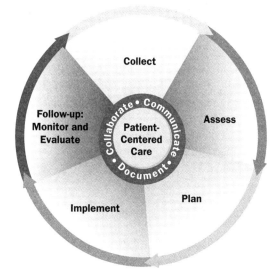

**Figure 1-5.** The Joint Commission of Pharmacy Practitioners Pharmacists' Patient Care Process.

# ■ PHARMACY DESIGN MODELS

## Pharmacy Design 101

There are numerous types of community pharmacies and many community pharmacies are uniquely designed. To set the stage for community pharmacy practice, it is important to understand various factors that are taken into consideration when designing the pharmacy. See Figure 1-6 for factors that impact the design of the pharmacy.

Before determining the design of the pharmacy, it is critical to review the state board of pharmacy regulations. Below are a few examples of state regulations that impact the design of the pharmacy:

- Pharmacy hours of operation
- Length and width of the pharmacy filling counter
- Access to running water, hot and cold
- Record-keeping requirements
- Dedicated space to offer patient care services

Some pharmacies are open anywhere from 8 to 12 h per day, while others operate 24 h per day to better meet patient needs. The prescription volume and hours of operation play a role in determining pharmacy staffing. Additionally, state boards of pharmacy have regulations that outline an allowable pharmacist to pharmacy technician ratio, and similarly there may be ratios for pharmacist to pharmacy interns or rotation students. Some pharmacies may operate under a pharmacy union contract. If so, the union contract may dictate the number of pharmacy employees that are required to work during a given shift and the

contract may include the maximum number of hours each pharmacy employee is allowed to work. Further detail on staffing is included in Chapter 3, "Human Resources Management."

One of the most important factors to consider when planning the design of the pharmacy space is pharmacy workflow. Pharmacy workflow should be efficient and optimize patient safety.[12] In general, workflow is the process of moving a prescription from the in-window where the patient drops off their prescription, through the required dispensing processes such as inputting the prescription, filling the prescription, verifying the prescription, and then to the out-window, where the patient picks up their prescription and received counseling. Workflow can be broken down into several workstations.[12] Examples of workstations include in-window, filling, pharmacist verification, and out-window.[12] See Figure 1-7 for an example of workflow workstations and activities conducted at each workstation and further information on workflow can be found in Chapter 3, "Human Resources Management" and Chapter 4, "Optimizing Pharmacy Workflow."

The pharmacy should be designed with adequate space for physical inventory, locked CII cabinet(s), storage of pharmacy supplies (e.g., prescription vials), refrigerator, freezer, and employee break area. If automation will play a role in the dispensing process, the pharmacy will need adequate space to house automated machines, such as storage or filling machines which may take up considerable space. The pharmacy may choose to sell over-the-counter (OTC) products, herbal products, and general merchandise. These products are typically stored outside of the pharmacy space, in a common area. The OTC, herbal and general merchandise sections should include popular items and items that the pharmacist routinely recommends. There may be some items preferably kept behind the counter such as nicotine replacement therapy and diabetes testing supplies as they are higher cost and warrant pharmacist counseling. The pharmacy should plan a defined space within the pharmacy to store products that may be sold without a prescription but must be sold behind the counter (e.g., pseudoephedrine, Plan B One-Step). These behind the counter products have additional

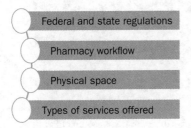

**Figure 1-6.** Factors impacting pharmacy design.

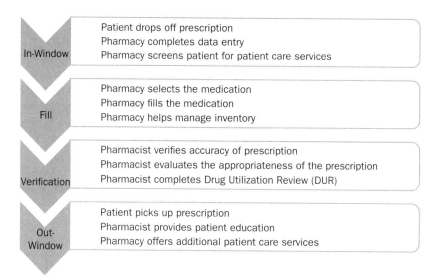

**In-Window**
Patient drops off prescription
Pharmacy completes data entry
Pharmacy screens patient for patient care services

**Fill**
Pharmacy selects the medication
Pharmacy fills the medication
Pharmacy helps manage inventory

**Verification**
Pharmacist verifies accuracy of prescription
Pharmacist evaluates the appropriateness of the prescription
Pharmacist completes Drug Utilization Review (DUR)

**Out-Window**
Patient picks up prescription
Pharmacist provides patient education
Pharmacy offers additional patient care services

**Figure 1-7.** Example workflow workstations and activities.

requirements the patient must meet in order for the pharmacy to be able to sell the product.

Another important component of designing a community pharmacy is to consider the types of services that will be offered at the location. Services may be offered to make the patient experience more convenient such as offering a drive-thru option for prescription pick up. If the pharmacy plans to offer medication delivery services for their patients, a space should be dedicated to preparing and shipping prescriptions orders. Another consideration is if the pharmacy is partnered with an assisted living facility that would need unit dose/blister packs. In this case, the pharmacy should design an area to prepare medications and assemble unit dose packets.

Additionally, the pharmacy design should include a space to offer patient counseling either in a private space or with a barrier to limit others from overhearing HIPAA sensitive information. Many pharmacies must also include a space to deliver patient care services such as immunizations, MTM, and travel health consultations. These patient care services may warrant a separate area or space, as these services may require more time and attention thus limiting pharmacy distractions is important. At the end of the day, the pharmacy should

be designed to ensure that the pharmacy remains organized and clutter free, which supports patient safety. The pharmacy design should allow for future growth and expansion as services change and grow.

As patient safety should be the priority of all pharmacy staff of a community pharmacy, one must be aware of all the resources available for continuous quality improvement. One such tool is the Medication Safety Self Assessment for Community/Ambulatory Care Pharmacy published by the Institute for Safe Medication Practices (ISMP).[13] This tool should be completed by a team of pharmacy owners/managers, staff pharmacists, pharmacy technicians, and pharmacy students to collaboratively assess the pharmacy systems by thoroughly investigating the level of implementation for each assessment item. This checklist allows the team to self-evaluate the pharmacy's processes for:

- Patient information
- Drug information
- Communication of drug orders and other drug information
- Drug labeling, packaging, and nomenclature
- Drug standardization, storage, and distribution
- Use of devices

- Environmental factors, workflow, and staffing patterns
- Staff competency and education
- Patient education
- Quality processes and risk management

The ISMP Medication Safety Self Assessment for Community/Ambulatory Care Pharmacy can be completed by any of the members of the pharmacy team, including pharmacy students and interns. If you are an intern or have an upcoming IPPE or APPE rotation in a community pharmacy, consider incorporating this tool. Your new perspective on the pharmacy's medication-use process and patient care services may help make important improvements to the pharmacy's safety and patient care. Even small and simple changes can make a big impact.

## Innovative Models

In the 1960s in Virginia, pharmacist Eugene White remodeled his drugstore from a typical pharmacy of the time, which included items such as a soda fountain and lunch counters to a professional office setting with a private consultation area, removed out-front merchandise and moved prescription product away from the patient's view.[3,14] Eugene White's pharmacy was the first model of its kind in the United States.[14] He introduced a paper chart based "Patient Record System" which is recognized as the first patient profile in pharmacy.[14] A prototype of White's model was introduced by then Vice President Hubert Humphrey at the 1965 APhA Annual Meeting, as the "Pharmaceutical Center" model.[3,14]

What was so revolutionary was at the time, the APhA's code of ethics did not support pharmacists discussing medication use with patients, and pharmacists did not work in partnership with physicians to promote the safe and effective use of prescription medications.[14,15] Eugene proposed the radical idea that pharmacists were better suited than physicians to answer patient questions about how prescriptions performed in the body.[14,15] Eugene White's pharmacy model became the basis for pharmacy consultation areas regularly seen in a modern pharmacy. The model helped set the stage for patient-centered care

and MTM, and deservingly, his pharmacy is preserved as a museum exhibit and classroom at Shenandoah University in Winchester, VA.[16]

Community pharmacies have continued to build and expand upon the example set by Eugene White. A study published by Willink and Isetts in 2005 detailed four patient-centered community pharmacies in Iowa and Minnesota: Iverson, Goodrich, Osterahaus, and Fairview Pharmacies.[17] The article described many common characteristics of these innovative pharmacies, including the physical environment design which was one of the most frequent questions these pharmacists received from their fellow colleagues.[17] Emphasis was placed on a professional and organized environment which empowers the patient and makes them feel secure and comfortable to share in-depth information about their medication-use behaviors.[17]

The patient-centered pharmacy environment typically employed the use of private and semi-private offices, booths, or spare rooms to assure patient confidentiality and provided a sense of trust and professionalism like White's Pharmaceutical Center model.[17] Interestingly, designated patient care areas, separate from patient care rooms, were often used in the pharmacies described in the article.[17] These patient care areas were designated counseling spaces that pharmacists used to discuss proper medication use and were separate from the dispensing and payment areas.[17] Physically separating the medication dispensing step and transactional nature of the payment area allows the patient and pharmacist to focus on the cognitive professional services being provided by the pharmacist.[17]

The Community Pharmacy Foundation (CPF) is a nonprofit organization dedicated to advancing community pharmacy practice and collaborative patient care delivery.[18] CPF is the founding sponsor of the Flip the Pharmacy (FtP) model. The Community Pharmacy Enhanced Services Network (CPESN®), USA, is a nationwide organization that represents individual, participating pharmacies that use evidence-based, patient-centered care.[19] On behalf of their pharmacies, CPESN® leverages the evidence-based, patient-centered care outcomes to reward the pharmacies for their performance. CPESN® and CPF

**Leverage the appointment-based model**

Medication Therapy Management (e.g., adherence)

**Improve patient follow-up and monitoring**

Schedule patient follow-up appointments

**Develop new roles for non-pharmacist support staff**

Work with pharmacy clerk/technicians on ways to support new services

**Optimize the utilization of technology and electronic care plans**

Document interventions in pharmacy system

**Establish working relationships with other care team members**

Develop and maintain relationships with other care team members, including those outside of the community-based pharmacy

**Develop business models and express value**

Utilize and establish payment models

**Figure 1-8.** Six transformation domains of Flip the Pharmacy..

have partnered to serve as the Coordinating Center for FtP.[19]

The FtP is a program designed to move community-based pharmacies business models from prescription-level care to providing longitudinal, patient-level care.[20] The goal is to prove the impact community-based pharmacies can have when offering longitudinal, patient-level care on a large scale, by incorporating numerous pharmacies.[20] The program offers practice transformation coaching to participating pharmacies to help them succeed.[20] Coaches develop a rapport with participating pharmacies and conduct on-site visits to provide insight and feedback on pharmacy workflow, patient care process, and business models. Six program domains have been identified and are supported by the transformation coaches.[21] See Figure 1-8. For more information on clinical services and CPESN, see Chapter 11, "Clinical and Value-Based Services."

## ▪ KEY TAKEAWAYS

Community pharmacy is a dynamic, ever-changing, environment. Understanding the history of community

pharmacy practice and pharmacy design will prepare you for the community pharmacy setting, whether it is your first day or you have been working there for years. Keys to success for a community pharmacy model include maintaining a clean, organized work environment, designing a physical pharmacy layout that promotes optimal dispensing and patient care services, and utilizing technology to make workflow more efficient. It is important for us to promote the advancement of community pharmacy by offering patient care services and establishing the pharmacists' role within the community. I challenge you to consider these questions as you advance in your pharmacy career. How do you see the role of the community pharmacist expanding in the future? How can you better prepare yourself for an advanced pharmacist's role in community pharmacy?

## ▪ CHAPTER APPLICATIONS

1. You are a pharmacy intern in the community pharmacy setting. A patient walks up to the counter and states that they have been started

on a new therapy that requires a healthcare professional to administer the medication to them every four weeks. The patient asks if the pharmacy can administer the medication so that they do not have to go to the provider's office for administration. You ask the pharmacy manager, and she confirms that medication administration is a service offered by the organization and is legal in the state; however, she is unfamiliar with the protocol. From the example chain organization chart, who in upper management would you contact to learn more about the medication administration service?

2. Provide examples of operational and patient care services that are routinely offered in the community pharmacy setting.

3. Provide examples of services that may be offered by a CPP.

4. The pharmacy is looking for ways to enhance the pharmacy experience so that it is more convenient for the patients. Due to the location and design of the pharmacy adding a drive-through window is not an option. What other type of service could the pharmacy offer to make the pharmacy experience more convenient for the patient?

5. The pharmacy hopes to free up the pharmacists time by automating a portion of the dispensing process. In addition to cost, what is the other factor that should be considered prior to determining the appropriate automation system.

# REFERENCES

1. American Institute for the History of Pharmacy (AIHP). Presentation A – Introduction to the Study of Pharmacy History. Madison, WI: AIHP; 2019. https://aihp.org/wp-content/uploads/2018/12/AACP-A.pdf

2. American Institute for the History of Pharmacy. AIHP Guidelines on Teaching History in Pharmacy Education. Madison, WI: AIHP; 2017. https://aihp.org/historical-resources/aihp-teaching-guidelines/

3. American Institute for the History of Pharmacy. Presentation B – Evolution of Pharmacy Practice. Madison, WI: AIHP; 2019. https://aihp.org/wp-content/uploads/2018/12/AACP-B.pdf

4. American Pharmacists Association (APhA). Vision and Mission for the Pharmacy Profession. Washington, D.C.: APhA; 2020. https://www.pharmacist.com/who-we-are#:~:text=APhA%20achieves%20our%20Mission%20by,recognition%2C%20differentiation%2C%20and%20leadership.&text=Raising%20societal%20awareness%20about%20the,care%20for%20optimal%20medication%20use. Washington, DC. June 2017. Accessed November 9, 2021.

5. Joint Commission of Pharmacy Practitioners (JCPP). JCPP Vision for Pharmacists' Practice. Alexandria, VA: JCPP; 2014. https://jcpp.net/resourcecat/jcpp-vision-for-pharmacists-practice/

6. Gallup website. Nurses continue to rate highest in honesty, ethics. https://news.gallup.com/poll/274673/nurses-continue-rate-highest-honesty-ethics.aspx Washington D.C. January 6, 2020. Accessed Sept 14, 2020.

7. Centers for Disease Control and Prevention. Get to know your pharmacist. Bethesda, MD: Centers for Disease Control and Prevention; 2018. https://www.cdc.gov/heartdisease/pharmacist.htm

8. Mazen Qato D, Zenk S, Wilder J, Harrington R, Gaskin D, Alexander GC. The availability of pharmacies in the United States: 2007-2015. *PLoS ONE.* 2017;12(8):e0183172. doi: 10.1371/journal.pone.0183172

9. Goode JV, Owen, J, Page A, Gatewood S. Community-based pharmacy practice innovation and the role of the community-based pharmacist practitioner in the United States. *Pharmacy (Basel).* 2019;7(3):106. doi: 10.3390/pharmacidy7030106

10. Bennett M, Goode JV. Recognition of community-based pharmacist practitioners: Essential health care providers. *J Am Pharm Assoc.* 2003;2016;56(5): 580-583. doi: 10.1016/j.japh.2016.04.566. Accessed November 9, 2021.

11. Joint Commission of Pharmacy Practitioners: Pharmacists' Patient Care Process. https://jcpp.net/wp-content/uploads/2016/03/PatientCareProcess-with-supporting-organizations.pdf Alexandria, VA May 20, 2014. Accessed September 14, 2020.

12. The Honest Apothecary. Retail Pharmacy Workflow Basics. http://www.thehonestapothecary.com/2014/07/17/retail-pharmacy-workflow-basics/. Whitinsville, MA July 17, 2014. Accessed November 9, 2021.

13. Institute for Safe Medication Practices: Medication Safety Self Assessment® for Community/Ambulatory Pharmacy. https://www.ismp.org/

assessments/community-ambulatory-pharmacy. Chicago, IL, January 3, 2017. Accessed November 9, 2021.

14. Higby GJ. The Continuing Evolution of American Pharmacy Practice, 1952–2002, *J Am Pharm Assoc.* 2002;42(1):12-15. doi: 10.1331/108658002763538017. https://www.sciencedirect.com/science/article/pii/S1086580215303181. Accessed November 11, 2021.

15. The Washington Post: Eugene White, 87, was 'revolutionary' of clinical pharmacies. https://www.washingtonpost.com/local/obituaries/eugene-white-87-was-revolutionary-of-clinical-pharmacies/2011/12/14/gIQA3HAwuO_story.html. Washington, DC, December 14, 2011. Accessed Sept 14, 2020.

16. Shenandoah University: Health Professions Building. https://www.su.edu/campus-maps/campus-locations/health-professionsbuilding/. Winchester, VA, June 4, 2020. Accessed September 14, 2020.

17. Willink DP and Isetts BJ. Becoming 'Indispensable': Developing Innovative Community Pharmacy Practices. *J Am Pharm Assoc.* 2005;45:376-89.

18. Community Pharmacy Foundation website. Vision and Mission. https://communitypharmacyfoundation.org/grants/vision.asp. Chicago, IL, 2020. Accessed November 9, 2021.

19. Community Pharmacy Enhances Services Network USA website. Commonly Asked Questions. https://www.cpesn.com/pharmacies/commonly-asked-questions/. Cary, NC, 2020. Accessed November 9, 2021.

20. Community Pharmacy Enhances Services Network USA. The Community Pharmacy Foundation Announces Flip the Pharmacy Practice Transformation Teams. https://www.cpesn.com/newsroom/the-community-pharmacy-foundation-announces-flip-the-pharmacy-practice-transformation-teams/#:~:text=Flip%20the%20Pharmacy%20aims%20to,use%20of%20hands%20on%20coaching. Cary, NC 2020. Accessed November 9, 2021.

21. Flip the Pharmacy website. Flip the Pharmacy homepage. https://www.flipthepharmacy.com/. Cary, NC, 2020. Accessed November 9, 2021.

# 2

# ENTREPRENEURSHIP AND INTRAPRENEURSHIP

*Kenneth C. Hohmeier, PharmD, and Raj Chhadua, PharmD, RPh*

## ▨ LEARNING OBJECTIVES

1.  Define key terms used for entrepreneurship and intrapreneurship.
2.  List the five skills of an innovator.
3.  Describe common methods used when planning for a new business venture.
4.  Describe the means by which one might finance a new venture or business.
5.  Define a junior partnership and describe when a pharmacist might consider this alternative financing model.

## ∎ SETTING THE SCENE

You are a community pharmacist at a busy chain pharmacy. Due to organizational restructuring and leadership turnover, your quality of work life has continued to decline. You continue to be asked to do more with less and your staff are slowly leaving for other opportunities. Patient complaints are on the rise, while your support from upper management continues to decline. However, the new pharmacy president brings an exciting new vision to the pharmacy and is looking for innovative solutions to boost profits and improve patient satisfaction. This initiative is asking for business proposals from pharmacists across the company, promising to fund the ideas with the most potential. You have several ideas you believe will work based on what you have seen from successful independent pharmacies in the area. You are presented with two options: stay at the pharmacy and help create a new business venture or "jump ship" to pursue the purchase of your own pharmacy from which you can launch your ideas.

## ∎ WHAT ARE ENTREPRENEURSHIP AND INTRAPRENEURSHIP?

Pharmacy is a dynamic industry and patient needs are constantly changing. Although this certainly can present feelings of uncertainty and stress, it also presents opportunity for those who have the best skills and ideas for the given moment. One hundred years ago, prior to the mass production of pharmaceuticals, industry and patient needs were centered on individual drug compounding. Fifty years later with the advent of the pharmaceutical industry, it shifted to managing drug interactions, larger manufactured inventories, and workflow. Today, in arguably the most rapidly changing time period in pharmacy, industry and patient needs center on convenience, cost, and the overall patient experience. The use of established principles of entrepreneurship and intrapreneurship allow pharmacists to use their unique experience and training to provide new and improved means to deliver patient care. It is impossible to know what future models of pharmacy practice will look like, but we do know it will be led by a group of innovative pharmacists who embrace these principles—and who, with perseverance and hard work, will lead the profession into the future.

### Entrepreneurship

The extraction of value through the introduction of new products or services, new means of production, or new organizational systems is known as *entrepreneurship*.[1] *Value* here is simply the difference between the worth of what you are offering your customers minus the cost of that offering. If the compounded medication you produce is worth $30 to a patient and your pharmacy can produce it for a cost of $25 then the value extracted is $5.

Defining entrepreneurship in this way ensures that one is not limited to the creation of a product or service to extract value from a system. A pharmacist may be entrepreneurial even without launching a new business, service, or product. For instance, in the pursuit of lowering the cost of compounding medications, a pharmacist might develop a new workflow method which centralizes all compounded medication fills to a single, centrally located pharmacy from which all compounds are then transported to all affiliated pharmacies within the organization. Using our earlier example, the cost of the compounded medication may decrease to $10/prescription; meaning that the extracted value for the pharmacy is now $20—a $15 increase per compounded prescription and boost to the pharmacy's "bottom line" even without selling anything new. The point here is entrepreneurship is not about a monocle-wearing capitalist building their monopoly so much as it is about offering a better product or service for a better price.

### Intrapreneurship

Related to entrepreneurship is the concept of *intrapreneurship*. Simply put, intrapreneurship is the use of entrepreneurial principles within an existing organization.[2]

As opposed to entrepreneurship, which is typically performed by individual business owners or top management teams (e.g., chief executive officers, company presidents), individuals at any level of the pharmacy organization may be intrapreneurial—from pharmacy technicians to staff pharmacists and pharmacy managers. This is of particular importance to the profession, as the number of independent pharmacies continue to decline, and as it becomes more difficult for independent pharmacies to compete in larger markets. Major examples of intrapreneurship include the launch of local employer-based vaccination programs by chain pharmacies (i.e., pharmacists onsite at an employer's office providing vaccines to employees over one or several days) and launching of point-of-care test-and-treat services for influenza and streptococcal pharyngitis.

There are several distinct differences between entrepreneurship and intrapreneurship. Entrepreneurial barriers may be largely external in nature and relate to financial planning, including break-even, cash flow, and raising of capital. Whereas, intrapreneurs are more likely to experience internal barriers, including resistance to change and managing the project's relative priority over other company priorities. Entrepreneurial facilitators may include newly formed companies and those with a smaller number of overall pharmacies that can be more nimble and able to quickly react to opportunities and threats. However, intrapreneurial ventures typically have the benefit of a team of seasoned leaders, an established financial model and more robust financial resources, and an established infrastructure from which to launch new projects.

Both entrepreneurship and intrapreneurship are financially beneficial for the pharmacy itself and the patients it serves. An organization which embraces and encourages intrapreneurship also has the added benefit of boosting engagement and productivity for frontline employees, according to recent research.[3]

## ▓ INNOVATION

At the foundation of both entrepreneurship and intrapreneurship is *innovation*. Innovation in community

pharmacy is the development of something new, such as a new approach, service, or product. Emerging research has identified the existence of several misconceptions around innovation. For example, just because something is innovative does not mean it is good. Innovation is also not limited to those things seen in news headlines (e.g., the iPhone®, Amazon®, Uber®). These innovations are referred to as *disruptive innovations*, and fundamentally alter an organization or even an entire marketplace. More commonly seen are *incremental innovations*, or significant improvements on existing products, processes, or services, but which do not themselves transform the pharmacy or the industry. Examples of incremental innovations include appointment-based medication synchronization and implementation of disease state management programs.

Most importantly there is the misconception that innovation is a rare trait for a few gifted individuals. While, in fact, innovation is not limited to random spurts of inspiration or to those who are blessed with creativity. Studies on identical twins have indicated that only about 25% of creativity is driven by genes; the remainder is due to our interactions with the world around us.[4,5] Furthermore, research supports the idea that innovation may be taught and the skill of innovating may be refined over time. This means that every pharmacist has the potential to be an innovator.

By practicing innovation skills used by top innovators, others may develop novel ideas. These skills are as follows:[5]

1. Associating: connecting seemingly unconnected ideas to form new ones
2. Questioning: asking "why" and "how" as often as possible before arriving at a solution
3. Observing: purposefully watching and noting the world around you to gain new insights
4. Experimenting: arriving at a new idea and then testing that idea as soon as possible, refining the idea, and testing again until the idea is refined into a workable prototype (try, fail, repeat)
5. Networking: seeking out interactions and conversations with individuals from different backgrounds and with different lived experiences then your own

Innovation may sometimes come as a spark of genius which is quickly jotted down on the back of a napkin, but more often innovation is generated proactively. There are several established tools which may be used for innovative ideas. These tools include:

1. Strengths, Weaknesses, Opportunities, and Threats (SWOT) analysis (see Chapter 11, "Clinical and Value-Added Services" for brief description)
2. Voice of the customer (methodically capturing the customer's expectations, needs, and dislikes)
3. Lean six sigma (see Chapter 4, "Optimizing Pharmacy Workflow" for brief description)

# PLANNING

## Lean Start-up

Often we think of launching new businesses or business opportunities as a large and formal effort requiring significant costs up front. However, a growing trend in entrepreneurial circles is the idea of the "Lean Start-up." The idea behind this methodology is for a business to invest the least amount of time and money in a new opportunity and only to meet the needs of early customers—being as *lean* as possible on costs and effort to reduce the risk on the organization. As all new ventures pose a significant burden on an organization in terms of tying up resources, a lean approach may be used to limit that burden while the pharmacy learns how to refine and perfect the new process, product, or service. This is opposed to spending time and money trying to perfect the new venture prior to its being launched, and hoping that it is what customers will want. An example of this may be an owner/operator working in a dual role as pharmacist and administrator.

## Business Model

All new business opportunities must, at some point, become financially viable—generating sufficient income to meet its financial obligations, including operating costs and debts at a minimum. Although financial management can be complex and does require consultation with financial experts, there are some basic

fundamentals of business planning which all pharmacists should be familiar.

The term *business model* is used to describe how the pharmacy plans to make money. More accurately, a business model is the assumption a company makes about why the company makes money. For instance, Amazon® was an online retailer for books, its original business model was as a retail bookseller. However, over time the organization's leadership realized that what it was being paid to do was provide customers with a quick, convenient, and user-friendly online marketplace. This "ah-ha" moment in Amazon®'s early years allowed it to expand into other areas of retail sales, and eventually into the pharmacy industry.

Developing a business model can be aided by the use of established business tools, similar to the process of innovation. One key tool used is the Business Model Canvas—a visual chart capturing several important factors in the development of a business model. These factors include:

1. Infrastructure: including key services and products for the pharmacy, available resources, and business partners including business alliances, wholesalers, buying groups
2. Offering: value proposition in terms of how the pharmacy will meet the needs of its patients (e.g., price, efficiency, patient satisfaction, patient outcomes)
3. Customers: who the pharmacy will serve, how relationships will be established and maintained, and how a pharmacy will attract new patients
4. Finances: how a pharmacy will make its money (e.g., prescription sales, over-the-counter sales, services, subscription fees)

## Business Plans

If your entrepreneurial or intrapreneurial idea requires raising funds you will likely be required to submit a *business plan*. A business plan is separate from a business model canvas, though many elements from the canvas may be incorporated into a business plan. The business plan is a formal written proposal for a new business or to make a major change to an existing one.[6]

Some key elements of a business plan include:

1. Executive summary
2. Business description
3. Products and/or services
4. Marketing analysis and plan
5. Operations and management
6. Financials
7. Conclusion

Business plans are a standard approach to garnering stakeholder support (e.g., bankers, loan officers, senior leadership); however, its popularity has begun to wane more recently.[8] In general, if the business venture is using an established business model with predictable variables in a stable industry, a business plan may still be the preferred approach. Opening, purchasing, or expanding a community pharmacy are classic examples of this as generally customer demand, distribution channels, costs, and industry trends have been stable over decades—even given the more recent shifts of third-party reimbursement models (i.e., direct and indirect remuneration fees, restricted pharmacy insurance networks). However, depending on the stakeholder and the specific idea, a truncated version of the business plan, known as a business case, may be preferred. For instance, if you are launching a new clinical service in a small independent pharmacy chain with five existing pharmacies, you may only need to develop a business case and pitch it to pharmacy ownership. A business case contains much of the same information as a business plan, but in a much more condensed format since the audience is likely to already have a good understanding of the pharmacy's existing mission and vision, strategic plan, and business model.

Some key elements of a business case include:

1. Executive summary: recommendation or plan, summary of solution
2. Introduction: business overview and key services, financial measures
3. Analysis: key assumptions, financial statements, costs
4. Conclusion: recommendations and next steps

Business planning runs the spectrum from more condensed briefings for stakeholders familiar with the pharmacy, such as a business case, to brainstorming innovative approaches to drive new business, such as the business model canvas, to a more formal business plan for a group of stakeholders with varying degree of knowledge about the pharmacy or pharmacy offering.

## Financing a New Venture or Business

Business ventures can be small or large, create new organizations or simply expand on existing ones, disrupt industries, or incrementally improve on existing services. Regardless of the *type* of venture, one thing ties them all together: money.

In the world of start-ups, this initial infusion of cash is often termed *capital* and may refer to both money and other assets available to an entrepreneur or organization, from which it has to start a new business venture. The level of detail necessary to raise capital varies depending on the idea in need of funding and the organization providing the funding. Generally, there are a few financing assessment basics with which entrepreneurs and intrapreneurs alike should be familiar. These are as follows:

1. Pro-forma cash flow statement: including capital requirements and start-up costs (see Chapter 8 on Profit, Loss, and Risk Management for more detail)
2. Pro-forma income statement and balance sheet (see Chapter 8, "Profit, Loss, and Risk Management" for more detail)
3. Break-even analysis: point at which total revenue equals total costs of the business; usually represented visually over time and the actual break-even point is where growing revenues exceed cost

These assessments are termed *pro forma*, Latin for "as a matter of form," because they are based on projections (i.e., estimates) of future business performance. This is opposed to cash flow statements, income statements, and balance sheets which are generated periodically for an existing business—which are not *pro forma*—and are based on actual and current financial accounting, rather than future projections. As the new venture does not have existing financial records, estimates are typically made based on industry benchmarks, such as NCPA's Community Pharmacy Start-up Benchmarking Report.[7]

## Estimation of Start-up Costs and Working Capital

A requirement of a thorough financial assessment is *start-up costs*, sometimes referred to as start-up capital. Some potential start-up costs include:

1. Cost of sales
2. Professional and consultative fees (e.g., legal, accounting, business consulting)
3. Technology (e.g., hardware, software, telephones, and security)
4. Operational costs (e.g., rent, pharmacy supplies, furniture)
5. Employee costs (e.g., salaries, payroll tax, benefits)
6. Marketing (e.g., promotional materials, advertising)

Start-up capital, including the initial costs of starting inventory, licenses, and equipment, are typically one-time expenditures meant to provide enough funding for a short period of time—typically around a year or two. Start-up costs can vary widely even among similar entrepreneurial ventures. Even if taking a lean start-up approach, it is advisable to build a cushion of 10–20% into your estimated start-up costs in anticipation of unexpected costs. For instance, a build-out of a new pharmacy may exceed what was budgeted. Or, unexpectedly high customer volume may require hiring of additional staff beyond what was initially estimated. These unanticipated costs must be covered by funds originally intended for other aspects of the start-up. This is the reason that one of the most common causes of business failure is undercapitalizing the start-up.

Beyond start-up capital, one must also consider *working capital*. Working capital is money available to cover the daily operations of the business (e.g.,

payroll, rent, inventory, supplies). This is particularly important in healthcare where third parties pay for a substantial amount of the services rendered (i.e., pharmacy benefit managers [PBMs] paying 80% of prescription drug price for the patient). Although the third party is contractually obligated to pay its share, payment may not be for 30, 45, or more days after services are rendered, depending on the contract. This may present a major strain on cash flow as pharmacies have to pay for inventory in a shorter timeframe and may be catastrophic in the long run if not considered. Once *pro forma* cash flow, income statements, and balance sheets have been completed, including a thorough estimation of start-up and working capital, one can pursue funding.

There are several sources for financing a new venture including:

1. Small business administration (SBA) loans
2. Venture capital and angel investors
3. Lines of short-term credit (e.g., credit cards)
4. Bank loans (conventional loan)
5. Home equity loans

Selecting the right source for funding should be based on thorough research and consultation with those with prior expertise when possible. However, there are some general rules for when to use each of these options. Lines of short-term credit, such as a business credit card, should be reserved for supplementing working capital, especially for times of fluctuating cash flow like around the New Year. Most entrepreneurs financing a pharmacy purchase or new pharmacy opening are eligible for SBA-guaranteed loans. The SBA does not loan money, but instead works with banks to provide the loan.[9] By the SBA partially guaranteeing payment on the loan, the lender has additional assurance that the loan will be paid even if the business venture fails. This allows a borrower to secure more favorable terms with less difficulty and with lesser required collateral or equity (e.g., assets including cash, property, or stakes in the business pledged to the lender by the borrower). Moreover, SBA loans can be stretched over 10–25 years as compared with conventional loans which range from 3 to 5 years. For entrepreneurs purchasing an existing pharmacy or building a new one, an SBA loan is an attractive option to finance the required loan of $500 000 to $1 000 000 as many entrepreneurs lack the collateral required to secure a conventional loan of that size.

Given that SBA loans are partially guaranteed by the SBA, applications can be tedious and overwhelming to those unfamiliar with the process. For those new to SBA loans, it is advisable to work with an SBA Preferred Lender Program to aid with the application and approval process.

Conventional loans are attractive options for those requiring less capital. Existing assets can be used as collateral to launch entrepreneurial or intrapreneurial ventures as part of an established business. However, start-ups will generally not be eligible for these loans. Conventional loans may be secured with lender collateral, or unsecured and reliant on the lenders credit history and established cash flow. Of the two, secured loans are the most common and less difficult to obtain since there is less financial risk on the part of the lender.

### Junior Partnerships

For many, the idea of owning and operating a pharmacy may seem out of reach. Raising capital and obtaining expertise are essential but intimidating prerequisites. One solution is a *junior partnership*—or the agreement of a lesser experienced pharmacist (junior partner) acquiring the pharmacy business from the more experienced pharmacist owner (senior partner) over a specified period of time. The key ingredient in a junior partnership is time itself. Time allows the junior partner to purchase larger shares of the pharmacy over the mutually agreed upon period of time—several years to several decades. Meanwhile, the senior partner provides guidance, support, and mentorship in the operations of the pharmacy over that same time period.

Regardless of the path you take to funding your entrepreneurial or intrapreneurial idea, there are plenty of resources and professionals who can and should guide you along the way. See Table 2-1 for a variety of

available resources. Beyond these resources, there are also numerous consulting groups who specialize in different areas of pharmacy practice. These groups can be found through internet searches, pharmacy conferences, and of course, networking with other pharmacists.

## ◼ OPERATIONAL CONSIDERATIONS FOR THE COMMUNITY PHARMACY ENTREPRENEUR

A thoughtful approach to your venture should include at the least the topics below. However, one should note that there is no "one-size-fits-all" or one "right" answer. Rather, one should aim not for what is "correct" but to instead aim for a robust understanding and conversation on each item. For instance, when thinking about location, an entrepreneur opening a new pharmacy should look at pharmacy locations in their region, reflect on their own pharmacy experience, ask patients, family, and friends for their needs around location, and speak with experts such as hired consultants, experienced or senior pharmacists, and pharmacy owners to get their thoughts.

*Location* within short proximity to customers is important for all successful businesses. However, in the pharmacy industry, location is especially critical—and poorly selected locations may sink an otherwise perfect business plan. One must consider access to highways and major roads—in terms of both proximity and traffic. For example, a pharmacy located on a busy road near a highway may seem perfectly located. However, if patients must turn left and cross the busy traffic to get to that pharmacy during rush hour it may in fact be a terrible location. In this case, locating the pharmacy for a right turn during rush hour may be better. A quick study of pharmacy locations around, you will likely find they occupy mostly corner locations, near traffic lights, and near high traffic areas. In general, 75% of the pharmacy's patients should be within 10 miles of the pharmacy—although in many areas of the country, it would not be unreasonable to target this within a 5-mile radius or less.

**Table 2-1. Resources for Pharmacist Entrepreneurs and Intrapreneurs**

| Organization | Website | Description |
|---|---|---|
| National Community Pharmacists Association (NCPA) | https://ncpa.org | NCPA provides a variety of useful resources and events for developing clinical services to launching new business. Their resources include consulting, books, advocacy, and even a "Pharmacy Ownership Workshop." |
| Live Oaks Bank | https://www.liveoakbank.com/pharmacy-loans/ | A small business lender, Live Oaks Bank, provides both resources and financial support. |
| McKesson | https://www.mckesson.com/Pharmacy-Management/Pharmacy-Ownership/ | McKesson is a drug wholesaler who offers a variety of resources to pharmacy owners. |
| Cardinal | https://www.cardinalhealth.com/en/services/retail-pharmacy/pharmacy-ownership.html | Cardinal is a drug wholesaler who offers a variety of resources to pharmacy owners |
| AmerisourceBergen | https://www.amerisourcebergen.com/solutions-pharmacies/independent-pharmacies | AmerisourceBergen is a drug wholesaler who offers a variety of resources to pharmacy owners. |
| American College of Clinical Pharmacy (ACCP) | https://www.accp.com/store/ | ACCP has a collection of resources and books to guide pharmacists. Topics range from starting a single clinical service to launching a brand new pharmacy. |
| Professional Compounding Centers of America (PCCA) | https://www.pccarx.com | PCCA is primarily a compounding pharmacy organization who provides resources for independent pharmacy owners. |

ACCP, American College of Clinical Pharmacy; NCPA, National Community Pharmacists Association; PCCA, Professional Compounding Centers of America.

*Workflow* is an important consideration in terms of safety and efficiency. Traditional pharmacy workflow steps include:

1. Data entry
2. Data entry verification
3. Product selection
4. Product selection verification
5. Product release to patient and counseling

These steps may vary from pharmacy to pharmacy, but generally use the following workflow principles:

1. Division of labor: focus on a single workflow step

2. Reduce waste: eliminate extra physical movement and task steps to reduce the time it takes to complete the task
3. Use of technology and automation: given enough task volume, use technology to aid in task completion
4. Continuous quality improvement: structured, proactive pursuit of better workflow processes

Technology for community pharmacy practice typically includes computer hardware and software (e.g., pharmacy software, barcoding, video conferencing software) and automation (e.g., dispensing robots, compounding machinery). Generally, technology allows for more efficient and safer care delivery—but this is not an absolute. In the early stages of a pharmacy start-up where prescription volume is low, the cost of some of these technologies may outweigh the benefits. For example, maintenance of automated dispensing robots may seem to reduce overall labor and increase workflow efficiency; however, such machines require significant maintenance to operate (e.g., troubleshooting errors, refilling machines with vials and medications) and may make more work for a pharmacy team with certain prescription volumes.

At its most basic level, a community pharmacy provides prescription products to a patient for the price of the drug, plus a fee. However, complexity is added when one zooms out and sees the pharmacy is in the middle of a larger supply chain which starts with the drug manufacturer and ends at the patient. Within this chain, there are wholesalers between the manufacturer and the pharmacy, and there are PBMs between the patient and the pharmacy. The pharmacy purchases medications from a pharmaceutical wholesaler, who, in turn, purchases the medications from the manufacturer. The PBM, or prescription insurance company, pays for medications on behalf of the patient. For this reason, pharmacies must carefully manage their relationships and contracts with these intermediaries (PBMs and wholesalers). The easiest way to do this is to join forces with other pharmacies and share resources, knowledge, and purchasing funds—and this is exactly what they do.

*Group purchasing organizations* (GPOs) are groups of pharmacies who partner to minimize costs by collectively negotiating contracts for things like medications. GPOs also work to maintain appropriate inventory levels and manage invoice payments. GPOs have continued to evolve over the years, and many now provide training and consultative services beyond medication purchasing into concepts like value-based reimbursement and data analytics.

Similar to GPOs, the *pharmacy services administrative organizations* (PSAOs) are groups of pharmacies who partner to collectively negotiate. In the case of the PSAO, these negotiations are related to PBMs and other third-party payers for reimbursement rates

and network access. PBMs represent over 90% of a pharmacy's total sales and so these negotiations are crucial to a pharmacy's financial success.

## SUMMARY

Entrepreneurship and intrapreneurship represent two pathways for pharmacists to improve overall quality of patient care and individual pharmacist job satisfaction. These paths often require a systematic approach to innovation to develop new means to provide value to patients and the pharmacy industry. New business ventures also require formal business planning. Fortunately, both innovation and business planning can be guided by principles and tools, and further facilitated by written and consultative expertise. Because pharmacy is a relatively stable business with predictable sales, financing a well-developed new pharmacy business plan is generally feasible, especially through SBA-secured lending. However, for some, it may be a better option to establish a junior partnership and slowly gain shares of the pharmacy, and expertise, over a longer period of time. Regardless of the type of venture you pursue as an entrepreneur or intrapreneur, planning for operations from the beginning will allow you enough time to solicit expert feedback and research different approaches. Although success is never guaranteed in business, thoughtful planning with input from trusted advisors and mentors can reduce risk and improve the odds for success.

## CHAPTER APPLICATIONS

1. At the beginning of this chapter (Setting the Scene), your pharmacy chain recently underwent significant structural changes. The result was not only a decrease in quality of work life, but also an exciting opportunity to join the new pharmacy president's vision. You can either leave the organization and pursue opening your own pharmacy or work with your existing employer

to launch new initiatives. List the two terms that best define each scenario and describe what each term means in your own words.

2. The decision in front of you to leave or stay with the pharmacy is one many pharmacists will face during their career. Using terms from the chapter, please compare and contrast the benefits and risks of each scenario. Which one would you choose? If you were 20 years further into your career would this change your mind?

3. Deciding to leave a company and pursue the opening of your own pharmacy can be a terrifying idea. However, a junior partnership has been suggested as a solution for those with limited experience and financial resources to enter into pharmacy ownership. Describe what a junior partnership is and how it differs from traditional entries into pharmacy entrepreneurship.

4. If you select to stay with the pharmacy you are currently employed at, you will need to begin working on some innovative ideas for the new president. What is innovation? Do you consider yourself innovative? Why? Is innovation something that is genetic or learned?

5. After weeks of waiting for a "spark" of innovation you are no further ahead in developing an innovative business idea for the pharmacy. Several other pharmacists have already pitched their ideas—and several feel that theirs will be selected for implementation. You are feeling the pressure. What are some structured strategies for creating the "spark" for innovation used by other highly effective innovators in different industries? List all five and how you plan on using them to create an innovative idea.

6. Several years later you decide that you want to put your experience and innovation skills "to the test" and open your own pharmacy. Given the rapid shifting of pharmacy practice over the years, you know that the way your pharmacy made money in the past is not how it will make money in the future. You decide to formally develop your business model. What is a business model? How can a business canvas help your business model and what are its primary components?

7. You have been gradually saving money for the new pharmacy by working at a chain community pharmacy for over 18 years and now have $75,000 which can be used for start-up costs. In addition, you are 15 years into a 30-year home mortgage which could give you another $150,000 in equity. Using terms from the chapter, describe what options are available to you for financing the pharmacy.

## REFERENCES

1. Chisholm-Burns M, Vaillancourt A, Shepherd M, Birtcher K. *Pharmacy Management, Leadership, Marketing, and Finance*. 2nd ed. Jones & Bartlett Publishers; 2012. Sudbury, MA.

2. Hohmeier KC, Gatwood J. Toward intrapreneurship in pharmacy education. *Am J Pharm Educ*. 2016 Apr 25;80(3).

3. Gawke JC, Gorgievski MJ, Bakker AB. Employee intrapreneurship and work engagement: a latent change score approach. *J Vocat Behav*. 2017 Jun 1;100:88-100.

4. Reznikoff M, Domino G, Bridges C, Honeyman M. Creative abilities in identical and fraternal twins. *Behav Genet*. 1973 Dec 1;3(4):365-377.

5. Dyer J, Gregersen H, Christensen CM. *The Innovator's DNA: Mastering the Five Skills of Disruptive Innovators*. Harvard Business Review Press; 2011. Boston, MA.

6. Zgarrick DP and Alston GL. *Pharmacy Management: Essentials for All Practice Settings*. 5th ed. McGraw Hill. 2019. New York, NY.

7. National Community Pharmacists Association. Community Pharmacy Start-up Benchmarking Report. Accessed January 1, 2021. http://www.ncpa.co/pdf/2020-ncpa-startup-report.pdf

8. Schramm C. It's not about the framework. Harvard Business Review. Published May–June 2018. Accessed January 1, 2021. https://hbr.org/2018/05/its-not-about-the-framework

9. Small Business Association. Accessed January 1, 2021. https://www.sba.gov

# 3

# HUMAN RESOURCES MANAGEMENT

*Jennifer Konieczny, PharmD, Megan Rhyne, PharmD, and Michelle Jeon, PharmD, BCACP*

---

## ▓ LEARNING OBJECTIVES

1. Identify strategies to conduct an effective interview and new hire selection.
2. Determine staff scheduling needs based on pharmacy-specific factors, such as prescription fill volume and services offered.
3. Describe a successful training program for various pharmacy team members including clerks, technicians-in-training, and certified pharmacy technicians.
4. Describe effective performance feedback methods for both pharmacists and technicians.
5. Recognize practical methods for handling conflict resolution in the pharmacy.

You have been a licensed pharmacist for 6 months and have just been asked by your regional supervisor to step into the role of pharmacy manager. With this new position, you will be relocating to a different pharmacy that has a high staff turnover rate and a reputation of a negative work environment. Your responsibilities include selecting and hiring a new technician, developing adequate training for him/her, and addressing staff performance issues that have been left unaddressed by the previous pharmacy manager. You have had minimal interaction with the staff thus far, and unfortunately cannot have an opportunity to consult with the previous manager since she is no longer employed by the company.

Regardless of job title and experience, all community pharmacists are expected to take part in personnel management activities. In the dispensing pharmacy, tasks must be prioritized and delegated, as the staff work together to provide efficient and quality care. Oftentimes, the pharmacist may be placed in charge of pharmacy technicians and student interns when the pharmacy manager is not physically present. Therefore, it is important for all pharmacists to learn and develop skills related to training, feedback, and conflict resolution. This chapter also provides insight into the fundamentals of interviewing and hiring, as well as labor management within a pharmacy.

# ■ INTERVIEWING AND HIRING STAFF

Interviews play a crucial role in the hiring process. It is often the quality of the interview that can have a considerable impact on the overall results of the hiring process. When interviewing candidates, you have a limited amount of time to cover all the information needed to decide if they are right for the position. Being prepared for an interview and implementing best-practice interview techniques can assist you in effectively and efficiently evaluating candidates and ultimately making the best hiring decision.

## Preparing for the Interview

Just as a candidate prepares for an interview, it is imperative that you as the interviewer are also prepared. Before the interview, you must review the candidate's application materials. This should include the candidate's licensing information (if required for the position), availability, work-related experience, and expected rate of pay. If you are hiring a pharmacist or a pharmacy technician, verify that they possess the required professional licensure with your respective state board of pharmacy, as you do not want to waste your time interviewing a candidate that is not qualified for the position. You may also want to check your state board's website for any prior disciplinary orders or actions that pertain to the candidate. While disciplinary orders do not immediately disqualify the candidate, it is something that should be discussed during the interview. It is also important to compare the candidate's listed days and times available to work with the scheduling needs of the pharmacy (e.g., opening/closing availability, willingness to work nights, weekends, holidays, other restrictions around school, family, and so on). When reviewing previous job experience for store clerk or pharmacy technician candidates, do not immediately disqualify those who do not have specific pharmacy-related experience. Previous experience in the retail sector can make a strong candidate for those who are familiar with providing customer service and working extended hours. Before conducting the interview, make sure you have clear expectations about what you are looking for in an ideal candidate for the respective position. It is especially helpful to prospective interviewees to include these expectations in the job listing and description (e.g., full-time vs part-time vs PRN, hours of availability, permanent vs temporary, language needs).

Prepare a list of questions to ask the candidate. These should include open-ended questions that are both behavioral and situational. Behavioral questions ask candidates to describe how they have handled past experiences. This allows you to get a glimpse into work ethic and ability to learn from difficult situations. Situational questions ask candidates to work through a hypothetical scenario that is relevant to the position. These questions allow you to assess the candidate's problem solving skills. Asking the right questions during the interview will help evaluate their competency in the field of pharmacy, willingness to learn and complete tasks, ability to handle tough customer situations, and ability to work well with others.

Refer to Figure 3-1 for sample interview questions.

## Starting the Interview

Many find interviews extremely stressful and may spend a lot of time preparing. To get an accurate sense of the candidate, it is important to provide a relaxed environment during the interview. Start by introducing yourself, making eye contact, and a simple pleasantry (e.g., "Thanks for coming in today to meet with me" or "It is so nice to meet you").

It is important to establish a rapport with the candidate. By establishing rapport, the candidate will be more open to answering questions thoughtfully and truthfully. Ask a few questions that will help you get to know the candidate as a whole and get the conversation started (e.g., "What made you want to get into pharmacy?" or "What drew you to a career in pharmacy?"). Once you have established rapport with the candidate, you can ease into the main interview so you may assess their qualifications for the position.

## Conducting the Interview

During the interview process, be sure to give the candidate plenty of time to reflect on the questions to

| Situational Questions | Behavioral Questions |
|---|---|
| How would you respond to a customer who is frustrated about how long it is taking to get their medication refilled? | Describe a situation where you worked as part of a team to finish a certain task. |
| If hired, how would you make sure that you get priority prescriptions filled in the right amount of time? | If asked, what would past coworkers say about you? |
| Describe how you would handle a situation where you've identified a medication error on a prescription that has already left the pharmacy. What would you do to resolve it? | Tell me about a time when you had to work closely with someone whose personality was different from yours. |
| *For a technician interview:* A patient comes to the pharmacy and requests a consultation about an over-the-counter medication, and the pharmacist is tied up on the phone. How do you handle this situation? | Have you ever worked with a coworker or manager that you either did not like or did not get along with? How did you handle that situation? |

Figure 3-1. Sample interview questions.

provide a well-thought-out answer. Take notes during the interview, listen to what they are saying, and evaluate their body language. If needed to make a better assessment of the candidate, encourage them to provide more detail by asking targeted follow-up questions. Do not be afraid of silence. If a candidate is struggling to answer a question, maintain silence to allow them to answer or for them to ask for clarification. Once you have completed your part of the interview, allow ample time for the candidate to ask any questions they may have. Their questions can be geared toward the company policies or specific pharmacy processes and procedures that you follow. Before the candidate leaves the interview, make sure you establish next steps (i.e., when they can expect to hear back from you, if a second interview is required, timeline for the hiring process, etc.).

Becoming an effective interviewer takes time and practice. Reach out to your store manager or human resources manager for help and guidance. When you conduct an effective interview, you will be able to assess the competency, experience, and personality of the prospective employee. This will help you to find the best fit for the needs of your pharmacy and team.

## ▦ STAFF SCHEDULE DEVELOPMENT

In order to run a pharmacy, you must be able to create a schedule based on labor needs. Having the right person at the right time in the right position is critical to maintain a successful pharmacy. Labor is a large operational cost and must be correctly managed to create and sustain a profitable pharmacy. Scheduling can not only impact labor costs, but employee morale and customer service as well.

### Labor Calculation and Determination

How labor is calculated or determined can change between employers. The overall result is that labor is controlled to fulfill prescriptions safely, completely, and at the lowest cost possible.

---

Weekly pharmacy sales = $85 000
Weekly total labor cost (10% of sales) = $8500
  ☐ Pharmacists (average $65/h x *80 h*) = $5200
  ☐ Technicians (average $15/h x *180 h*) = $2700
  ☐ Clerks (average $10/h x *60 h*) = $600
*\* Hours will vary to meet demand and total labor cost*

**Figure 3-2.** Percentage of sales example.

Here are some examples of how companies may determine labor cost goals:

- *Percentage of sales*, e.g., total labor cost is expected to remain below 10% of total sales. This is accomplished by knowing the average labor cost for each job category in the pharmacy and calculating the total weekly hours associated with those categories. The amount of hours can be manipulated to total the weekly labor cost driven by weekly sales. See Figure 3-2 for example.
- *Weekly script volume*, e.g., a pharmacy is expected to fulfill 2 360 scripts/week to cover the cost of labor. The cost of dispensing can be translated into how many scripts equate the labor of one technician hour. For example, if a pharmacy is filling fewer scripts than budgeted, technician hours are cut to account for the loss in revenue to cover labor costs. See Figure 3-3 for example.

Most employers will have training about how to execute a schedule based on the requirements they use to develop schedules. It will be your responsibility to ensure your schedule is executed and monitored on a weekly basis.

### Scheduling Execution

Creating an effective schedule can be intimidating and time consuming; it is much like piecing together a complex puzzle. It requires a balance of anticipating the needs of your customers, the needs of your staff, and the job duties that must be completed. A scheduling template has been provided to assist you with this process (see Table 3-1). Use this template while

13 prescriptions = 1 technician hour

| Day | Budget | Actual | Difference | Tech Hours |
|-----|--------|--------|------------|------------|
| 1 | 150 | 140 | −10 | |
| 2 | 125 | 120 | −5 | |
| 3 | 460 | 450 | −10 | −1 h |
| 4 | 490 | 515 | +25 | |
| 5 | 400 | 385 | −15 | |
| 6 | 360 | 340 | −2 | −1 h |
| 7 | 375 | 380 | +5 | |
| Total | 2360 | 2330 | −30 | 2 h |

In the example above, after Days 1 and 2, the pharmacy is short by 15 h, so on Day 3 you cut 1 technician hour. Day 4 is strong, but Day 5 script volume drops again, and so on Day 6 another technician hour is removed from the schedule. At the end of the week, you have reduced 2 technician hours to account for the loss in script volume.

**Figure 3-3.** Weekly script volume example.

completing the following steps to make an effective schedule.

Step 1: Start with the total amount of hours the pharmacy is open each day. Be sure to adjust for holiday hours as needed.

Step 2: Determine the amount of hours to be used for each staff type (pharmacist, technician, clerk, and intern). This may be provided by your employer or calculated according to predetermined metrics.

Step 3: Input staff availability. This is an important step to ensure you do not schedule a staff member when they are not available.

Step 4: Schedule pharmacist shifts. The pharmacist schedule is usually a set of 2- or 3-week rotating schedule that is fair and equal. Schedule overlap, if available, during busiest days so prescription volume and sales reflect labor usage accordingly. Pharmacist mealtime or breaks should be considered if permitted by the company. Pharmacist labor is the highest labor cost on the payroll, so it must be justified and used appropriately.[1]

Step 5: Schedule technician shifts. Schedule for workflow as well as non-workflow duties, such as putting away the order or completing medication therapy management (MTM) calls. Assign shifts to technicians based on skill and availability. You should take into account the strengths and weaknesses of your staff and place them appropriately according to the demands of the pharmacy. Ensuring the correct technician opens or closes can affect the workflow for the rest of the day if not scheduled correctly. Be sure to schedule technicians fairly and rotate opening, closing, and midday shifts. Technicians can be full-time or part-time employees, so make sure you are providing the required number of hours to maintain their employment status. As hourly wageworkers, breaks must also be accounted for when scheduling technicians.

Step 6: Schedule clerks, if available. Clerks have other duties as well as checking out customers, such as placing completed prescriptions into the waiting bin or putting away an order. However, the customer-facing interaction is the most important component of their role. Use your metrics to determine peak register times to schedule clerks accordingly. Similar to technician schedules,

**Table 3-1.  Staff Scheduling Template**

| Hours | Monday | Tuesday | Wednesday | Thursday | Friday | Saturday | Sunday | Total |
|---|---|---|---|---|---|---|---|---|
| **Pharmacist** | | | | | | | | |
| RPh1 | Shift | Shift | Shift | Shift | Shift | Shift | Shift | |
| RPh2 | Shift | Shift | Shift | Shift | Shift | Shift | Shift | |
| | | | | | | | Budget Hours | Actual Hours |
| **Technician** | | | | | | | | |
| Tech 1 | Availability / Shift | Availability / Shift | Availability / Shift | Availability / Shift | Availability / Shift | Availability / Shift | Availability / Shift | Total Hours / Tech 1 |
| Tech 2 | Availability / Shift | Availability / Shift | Availability / Shift | Availability / Shift | Availability / Shift | Availability / Shift | Availability / Shift | Total Hours / Tech 2 |
| Tech 3 | Availability / Shift | Availability / Shift | Availability / Shift | Availability / Shift | Availability / Shift | Availability / Shift | Availability / Shift | Total Hours / Tech 3 |
| Tech 4 | Availability / Shift | Availability / Shift | Availability / Shift | Availability / Shift | Availability / Shift | Availability / Shift | Availability / Shift | Total Hours / Tech 4 |
| | | | | | | | Budget Hours | Actual Hours |
| **Clerk** | | | | | | | | |
| Clerk 1 | Availability / Shift | Availability / Shift | Availability / Shift | Availability / Shift | Availability / Shift | Availability / Shift | Availability / Shift | Total Hours / Clerk 1 |
| Clerk 2 | Availability / Shift | Availability / Shift | Availability / Shift | Availability / Shift | Availability / Shift | Availability / Shift | Availability / Shift | Total Hours / Clerk 2 |
| Clerk 3 | Availability / Shift | Availability / Shift | Availability / Shift | Availability / Shift | Availability / Shift | Availability / Shift | Availability / Shift | Total Hours / Clerk 3 |
| | | | | | | | Budget Hours | Actual Hours |
| **Intern** | | | | | | | | |
| Intern 1 | Availability / Shift | Availability / Shift | Availability / Shift | Availability / Shift | Availability / Shift | Availability / Shift | Availability / Shift | Total Hours / Intern 1 |
| Intern 2 | Availability / Shift | Availability / Shift | Availability / Shift | Availability / Shift | Availability / Shift | Availability / Shift | Availability / Shift | Total Hours / Intern 2 |
| | | | | | | | Budget Hours | Actual Hours |

ensure that clerks are scheduled fairly and with appropriate breaks.

Step 7: Schedule pharmacy student interns, if available. Interns can be difficult to schedule due to their school schedule demands. Some companies require a minimum number of hours to be worked each week to keep an intern active on the payroll. Weekends are common times interns are scheduled, but keep availability open during the week as well to assist the pharmacist during busy times in the morning or evening.

Step 8: Verify legal requirements are accounted for while making the schedule. These legal requirements include pharmacist to technician ratio, pharmacist to intern ratio, required breaks after a certain amount of time worked, etc.

Step 9: Once the first draft of the schedule is complete, review to ensure tasks and customer-facing activities are properly accounted for and scheduled for. These tasks include, putting up orders, MTM services, and ensuring enough staff to cover busy pickup times. Also, confirm whether scheduled shifts align with staff availability.

Step 10: Complete a final check to verify scheduled hours align with budgeted hours.

## Scheduling Considerations

To ensure the schedule is adhered to by pharmacy staff, there are a few situations you should avoid. The first issue is avoiding overtime (OT). OT can significantly affect your labor budget as employees are paid at a higher rate, usually time and a half after working 40 hours, which significantly cuts into pharmacy profit. A best practice to prevent OT is to schedule staff at 39.5 hours, which allows for fluctuations during shifts, when appropriate. This is also helpful to avoid having to cut hours later in the week to ensure OT is not accrued. As a pharmacist, it is your responsibility to ensure the schedule is being followed by all staff, including clocking in and out on time and ensuring staff are taking shift breaks. If staff are not taking scheduled breaks at the correct time, it can cause

unnecessary service or workflow issues. Lastly, you may need to reduce hours based on lower than anticipated prescription volume or sales, commonly referred to as flexing down time. Flexing down time can be challenging but not impossible. Daily tracking of prescription volume or sales is the best way to account for reductions in pharmacy revenue and anticipate the need to flex down labor. If determined that flexing down is necessary, take into account the needs of the pharmacy during the next shift or business day and adjust accordingly. For example, if you need to flex down on Friday, but know that Friday evening is busy in the pharmacy, ask technicians to come in late or take extended lunch breaks instead of leaving early.

Another important part of scheduling is having contingency plans during illness or vacation. Staff that have additional availability from their current schedule can be used when another staff member calls in sick or requests vacation. This allows you to utilize your own staff as opposed to borrowing staff from other stores, if part of a chain. If your staff is already working their availability and allowed hours, you may be able to reach out to neighboring stores for assistance. A best practice is to reach out to the other pharmacy manager(s) to inquire about technicians who might be available to help your store, stating specific days and times of needed help. Flexibility with your schedule may be necessary to work around other stores' availability and staff. Planning vacations is important and requires communication with your entire staff. Creating a community pharmacy calendar is another best practice to ensure that staff and scheduler are aware of time off and vacation requests. This calendar can also be helpful for staff to know which weekends they will be working if on a rotating schedule. Proper planning and contingency plans are important to keep workflow as normal as possible during staff absences.

Scheduling demands can fluctuate during the week, month, or year. Use company metrics to help determine peak pickup times, heavy prescription input and busy dispensing times, as well as other tasks in the pharmacy during the week. Fridays can be busy pickup days because many people receive their paychecks;

Mondays are often busy with an influx of refill authorizations and trips to the provider's office after the weekend; and days you receive inventory replenishment orders will take staff away from workflow duties. By anticipating these increases in business and tasks, you can schedule enough staff to check out customers and fill prescriptions effectively. Metrics can also be used to determine fluctuations during the month. Depending on the pharmacy's demographics, the first of the month can be a busy time when customers receive social security, disability, or other forms of income and can afford to pick up their prescriptions; therefore, more staff will be needed to fill and check out customers. The time of year will also change the amount of support staff needed to keep the pharmacy operating smoothly. During colder months, script volume tends to increase because of more infection and the need for more prescriptions. Immunizations also peak during flu season, diverting staff from dispensing duties to vaccination duties, including entering, processing, and delivering vaccines to patients. Conversely, it is important to understand that script volume and sales may decrease during summer months, so less staff will be needed in the pharmacy. Employers measure many aspects of the pharmacy; therefore, it is your duty to review and utilize this information to maintain a well-operating pharmacy.

A growing part of community pharmacy is the incorporation of MTM services to mitigate Direct and Indirect Remuneration (DIR) fees. MTM services should be a priority to all pharmacy managers in order to avoid costly DIR fees. A best practice is to include MTM services into daily workflow by both technicians and pharmacists. Budget time during mid-morning and evening times to reach customers and complete the services, instead of missing opportunities to bill completed cases. When making a schedule, review the MTM platform your company uses to assess how much time will be committed to MTM services and schedule accordingly. Make certain your staff is aware of the tasks required, so this dedicated time is utilized appropriately. Adherence calls, which take about 5–15 min to complete, should be made when they are most likely

to be effective by reaching the customer (e.g., elderly retired patients may be called in the mornings, working patients should be called in the evenings). Comprehensive medication reviews (CMRs) are a large and time-consuming component of MTM services that are very important to insurance contracts and performance ratings. CMRs can take 45–60 min to complete. The preparation of the CMR should be completed during less busy times in the pharmacy, such as during weekends. It is important to schedule time to conduct a CMR with a patient during pharmacist overlap hours or when the pharmacist can be removed from workflow for an extended time. Utilizing pharmacy interns for CMRs is also helpful for both the preparation and delivery of CMRs. CMRs prepared and conducted by interns should always be done with pharmacist supervision.

Workstation assignment boards (see Table 3-2) are one popular tool pharmacies will use to ensure staff are aware of tasks that need to be completed and where in the workflow they should focus. A workstation assignment board is a tool visible to all staff that breaks down specific times during the day and lists specific tasks to be performed by an assigned staff member. This can be advantageous so that staff do not get overwhelmed by the pharmacy workload demands, and helps them to focus on a certain task or point of workflow to ensure things get completed harmoniously. A basic board includes workflow stations such as data entry, pickup, product dispensing, verification, and drive-thru window, as well as tasks outside of workflow such as breaks, MTM services, inventory duties, schedule development, or cleaning.

Managing labor is a critical role of the pharmacist in community pharmacy. Execution of a well-made schedule is important to ensure all tasks and duties are completed by the staff, while keeping labor costs manageable. Maintain consistent communication with your staff to ensure their satisfaction and solicit input about altering the schedule as demands change. For additional information on how to optimize workflow, see Chapter 4, "Optimizing Pharmacy Workflow."

**Table 3-2. Workstation Assignment Board Example**

| Time | Pharmacist | Technician | Clerk | Break | Duties |
|---|---|---|---|---|---|
| 8–9 AM | RPh1: Verification | Tech1: Data Entry Dispensing | Clerk 1: Pick-up Drive-thru | | |
| 9–10 AM | RPh1: Verification | Tech1: Data Entry Tech2: Dispensing | Clerk 1: Pick-up Drive-thru | | |
| 10–11 AM | RPh1: Verification | Tech1: Data Entry Tech 2: Dispensing | Clerk 1: Pick-up Clerk 2: Drive-thru | | Tech 3: Inventory (receive order) |
| 11–12 PM | RPh1: Verification | Tech1: Data Entry Tech 2: Dispensing | Clerk 2: Pick-up Drive-thru | Clerk 1: Lunch | Tech 3: MTM calls and platform review |
| 12–1 PM | RPh1: Data Entry RPh2: Verification | Tech 3: Dispensing Tech 2: Dispensing | Clerk 2: Pick-up Clerk 1: Drive-thru | Tech 1: Lunch | |
| 1–2 PM | RPh2: Verification | Tech 3: Data Entry Tech 2: Dispensing | Clerk 1: Pick-up Drive-thru | Clerk 2: Lunch | RPh1: Schedule |
| 2–3 PM | RPh2: Verification | Tech 3: Data Entry Tech 1: Dispensing | Clerk 1: Pick-up Drive-thru | Tech 2: Lunch | RPh1: CMR Clerk 2: Cleaning |
| 3–4 PM | RPh1: Data Entry RPh2: Verification | Tech 2: Dispensing Tech 1: Dispensing | Clerk 2: Pickup Drive-thru | Tech 3: Lunch | |
| 4–5 PM | RPh2: Verification | Tech 2: Data Entry Tech 1: Dispensing | Clerk 2: Pickup Clerk 3: Drive-thru | | Tech 3: MTM calls |
| 5–6 PM | RPh2: Verification | Tech 2: Data Entry Tech 3: Dispensing | Clerk 2: Pickup Clerk 3: Drive-thru | | |

*(Continued)*

**Table 3-2. Workstation Assignment Board Example (*Continued*)**

| Time | Pharmacist | Technician | Clerk | Break | Duties |
|------|-----------|-----------|-------|-------|--------|
| 6–7 PM | RPh2: | Tech 3: | Clerk 3: | | Tech 2: |
| | Verification | Data Entry | Pickup | | Inventory (place order) |
| | | Dispensing | Drive-thru | | |
| 7–8 PM | RPh2: | Tech 3: | Clerk 3: | | |
| | Verification | Data Entry | Pickup | | |
| | | Dispensing | Drive-thru | | |

## ■ STAFF TRAINING STRATEGIES

### Initial Training

Before training a new employee, you must first establish the procedures and expectations of the training process. Set realistic goals by building upon the employee's current skill level and experience. Check with your employer to see if they have training procedures or guidelines, and determine if training hours are allotted for scheduling purposes. Although all new employees will need to follow company-specific training guidelines, experienced technicians and pharmacists will require less one-on-one training time. Make sure to check-in with your new employee regularly during their first few weeks to assess knowledge and possible areas for retraining. Here are a few initial steps to follow when training a new employee:

1. Review training outline or guidelines to establish timeline and goals.
2. Review job roles and responsibilities.
3. Introduce new employee to team.
4. Conduct pharmacy tour to describe layout and workstations.
5. Complete onboarding checklist with trainer.

### Continuous Training

The pharmacy industry is constantly changing, requiring employers and employees to adapt. Many companies offer e-learning training modules to be completed on a regular basis. They can be monthly updates or even yearly recertifications for required training such as:

- Medicare Fraud, Waste, and Abuse
- Combat Methamphetamine Epidemic Act
- Health Insurance Portability and Accountability Act
- Bloodborne Pathogens
- Safe Disposal of Hazardous Wastes

A challenge with experienced technicians can be a lack of engagement and the stagnant feeling of performing the same tasks every day. Since pharmacy is constantly changing, placing experienced technicians in charge of new processes or training can improve their engagement. Incorporating experienced technicians into the training of new staff or soliciting feedback to optimize pharmacy operations can also improve their satisfaction with their job duties.

### Retraining

There may be times in the pharmacy when your staff is in need of retraining because of workflow, safety, or service issues. If a technician is struggling at a specific workstation, it is important to help develop that technician and not allow them to avoid their deficiencies. Allow the technician instead to work that station at slower times, so they do not feel as pressured, or partner with another technician so they can feel comfortable asking questions and can gain insight to best practices to be proficient at that station. If your staff are making mistakes that lead to safety issues such as incorrectly typed prescriptions at data entry, placing incorrect tablets into dispensing vials, or selling prescriptions to the incorrect patient, retraining and reviewing pharmacy processes must occur. Continuing education courses are available through various sources such as, *Pharmacist's Letter,* state board of pharmacy websites, and schools of pharmacy. Your employer may also have a retraining program to ensure staff is reducing the amount of medication errors in the pharmacy. If you have staff who are struggling with service-related issues with customers or colleagues, a one-on-one intervention may be necessary. Teaching "soft skills" can be challenging, as some companies do not offer any training in this area. Resources are available to aid in how to discuss issues and deal with stressful situations with staff, which will be discussed later in this chapter.

## Training Challenges and Potential Solutions

Challenges may arise during the training process. First, your pharmacy may experience a situation where there are a large number of minimally experienced technicians at one time. One solution to that problem is to swap technicians with another pharmacy that has many experienced technicians, who can both help train and keep the workflow running efficiently in your pharmacy. This also allows the new technicians to see how a well-trained pharmacy operates, and gives them time with "experts" in their profession who can provide best practices and helpful hints for resolving issues correctly and quickly.

Another issue may be the feeling there is not enough time to train a new employee. Training usually requires a certain amount of time regardless of experience or learning style. Some new hires may require more help than others, but it may seem impossible with real-time demands of the pharmacy. In this situation, utilize less busy times and days of the week such as weekends to schedule more one-on-one time with an experienced technician. Building confidence in a newly hired employee is important and requires time investment to develop their skills so they can function independently.

## ◼ PROVIDING EFFECTIVE PERFORMANCE FEEDBACK

Oftentimes, the responsibility of delivering feedback can be perceived as a manager's duty. However, even pharmacists without managerial roles have countless opportunities to utilize these same tools to optimize a positive and effective work environment.

Feedback can be categorized into two types: formative and summative. Formative feedback is given on a more frequent basis, and is used to help elicit positive change or improvement in a team member. Summative feedback is typically given annually, and often provides a formal evaluation to justify a raise, bonus, or disciplinary action. On-demand formative feedback can be delivered by anyone and is most useful when applied on at least a daily basis.

## When to Provide Feedback

In the community pharmacy setting, the method of delivery and timing of feedback that is given can be very important. If related to a specific task or patient encounter, either positive or constructive feedback is most effective when given on the spot. For example, you notice that a pharmacy technician working with you handled a particularly difficult patient well. A simple feedback statement such as, "I think you did a great job keeping a positive attitude and staying patient during that phone call" immediately after the phone call is often appreciated, and encourages that behavior for future patient encounters.

On the other hand, if feedback is needed to comment on a skill or characteristic observed more than once, it may be best to wait until the end of the day or week to have an opportunity for discussion, if needed. For example, you may notice a new pharmacy intern has consistently displayed unprofessional behavior throughout the day, such as making rude comments about patients after they leave the pharmacy. By the end of the day, you realize that this behavior will likely continue if unaddressed. It would be best to pull this intern aside before he/she leaves for the day, to bring attention to this trending behavior early. At the same time, it would be important to make sure this feedback is provided in a private setting, so the intern does not feel embarrassed in front of others.

Even constructive feedback can be delivered on the spot, if immediate action is needed. An effective pharmacist should not hesitate to communicate often and truthfully. For example, a pharmacy technician makes a mistake entering a prescription, and you catch the error. Take a moment to explain the error and ask him/her to fix it, immediately.

Pharmacists who may be new to the pharmacy or the role might attempt to avoid this potential confrontation, and instead choose to fix the error themselves quietly. Over time, this type of evasive behavior can lead to two major issues. First, the pharmacist does not share the burden of preventing similar future mistakes within workflow, which may increase the chance of a medication error occurring. This ultimately can result in patient harm, as a direct result of lack of communication and ineffective teamwork. The second issue is that if the team member is unaware of the problem(s), he/she does not have the opportunity to improve. When the time comes for summative feedback, in the form of an annual evaluation or formal warning, the conversation can result in shock or confusion. At this point, a positive work relationship may be in jeopardy, due to a perceived loss of trust.

## How to Provide Feedback

It can be difficult to recognize areas to provide positive feedback, compared to negative feedback in a pharmacy setting. Pharmacists often are in the mindset of identifying and resolving problems, whether it is when checking a prescription or educating a patient. As a result, if the pharmacist does not make a conscious effort to acknowledge positive behaviors in their team members and only verbalizes negative feedback when necessary, technicians and fellow pharmacists may feel underappreciated or may feel they are not meeting expectations. There are several methods that can be utilized to provide effective feedback.

One strategy is called the sandwich method.[2] This method is when a criticism is "sandwiched" by two positive comments of praise. This strategy may be useful when the relationship between the feedback giver and recipient is not yet well established, or when you wish to offset the potentially negative reaction to the criticism. The "buns" of the sandwich provide context to the presented criticism, and allow the recipient to identify ways to hone their skills. For example, "I appreciate your efficiency when completing tasks, because it makes workflow move very quickly." *(Praise)* "However, I noticed that the errors that you tend to make are due to a lack of attention to detail. For example, you entered a prescription under the wrong patient with a similar name today." *(Criticism)* "I encourage you to slow down and double check your work. Since you're a quick learner and dedicated worker, you'll get quicker naturally over time." *(Praise)*

Characteristics of good feedback include sincerity, specific examples, suggestions, and an opportunity to respond. Be sure to give feedback, whether positive or negative, sincerely. This applies to both the words that are spoken and the body language that accompanies it. It is not helpful or effective to give half-hearted feedback, even if it is positive. Feedback also should always include specific examples, to illustrate how the team member has demonstrated a perceived characteristic. For example, if you tell a student intern, "You're so good at giving immunizations!," the intern likely will not have a clear idea of what exactly is being done well. Instead, provide examples such as, "The way you kept Ms. Jones's vaccine doses and paperwork organized when she wanted three vaccines at once was very impressive," to give robust substance to the observation.

If a team member requires constructive feedback, including suggestions for improvement is often necessary. This allows the recipient to see a potential pathway to meet expectations, rather than concentrate on what was done incorrectly. For example, a pharmacy technician who has been working with you for several weeks now, continues to ask you the same questions each week about how to check in the pharmacy order. A sub-optimal way to deliver this feedback would be, "You've asked me this question for the third time now. Do you not remember what I told you last week?" An approach such as, "I've noticed that you've needed help remembering the process for checking in the order for the last few weeks now. I suggest you write down the steps in a notebook today, so you can refer to it next time and eventually commit it to memory" would be more likely to elicit positive change.

The final characteristic to consider is providing the recipient an opportunity to respond to feedback. Ideally, formal feedback discussions, such as a quarterly evaluation, should be a two-way conversation to allow both parties to provide their observations. Be sure to ask open-ended questions during feedback sessions to clarify or explain motivations or intent. The ultimate goal is to mutually agree on a plan to improve behaviors if needed, or to maintain a high quality of care.

## Additional Feedback Considerations

Supervisors must remember to document all formal feedback properly, whether it is verbal or written. According to site-specific policies, disciplinary action may not be able to be taken unless certain procedures involving feedback have been followed. Some pharmacy businesses may implement a performance improvement plan, which is a structured approach to give employees who are not meeting expectations an opportunity to succeed with monitoring. It is extremely important to keep record of when (date and time) formal feedback was delivered, and what was discussed during each encounter. This provides third-parties, such as the Human Resources department, a more comprehensive view of what may ultimately lead to disciplinary action.

If a team member does require major improvements that may take time to fully address, an effective supervisor should ensure that the employee is consistently aware of where they stand in the disciplinary process. Even if the first step is to give a formal verbal warning, it should be made clear during the conversation that the verbal warning will be documented and can progress to additional measures. An employee should never feel blindsided because it was not explicitly made clear that prior feedback was documented as formal warnings.

Supervisors should also be sure that proper escalation of disciplinary action is followed, so all employees are treated equally. Unless stated in site policies for extenuating circumstances, incremental steps generally should not be skipped when implementing disciplinary action.

## ■ CONFLICT RESOLUTION

As workplaces usually employ a diverse staff, there will undoubtedly be situations where work ethic, personalities, and communication styles do not mesh well between coworkers. Although the optimal goal is to create and maintain a positive environment with minimal conflict or tension, sometimes this is not possible. As a pharmacist and leader of workflow, it is important to maintain the focus required to provide quality patient care to our customers. If this primary objective is not being met as a result of personnel conflict, intervention is required.

Avoiding conflict is a natural tendency for many people. It is important to identify when conflict is developing and how to defuse it. A trap many supervisors may fall into is the notion that silence is perceived as acceptance. Just because an issue isn't explicitly brought to your attention, doesn't mean it will always resolve itself without intervention. Once a conflict is identified, the pharmacist should aim to address it immediately.

Emotional intelligence is a significant component of resolving conflict. Emotional intelligence is the ability to identify your emotions and the emotions of others and manage them appropriately.[3] When resolving conflict, it is important for you to evaluate and recognize your emotions during a situation and ensure they do not drive your decision making in a negative way. If you are feeling frustrated at a person or situation, take a minute to evaluate what is causing and what might relieve that frustration. It is also important to understand how others are feeling so you can help them understand how to turn those emotions into something positive. By taking a step back and evaluating the emotions involved, it is easier to resolve the conflict.

If there is a conflict between support staff and the pharmacist, it is the pharmacist's responsibility to remedy the situation. The longer a conflict goes unresolved, the more tension may build and become apparent to fellow coworkers and customers. Meeting one-on-one is necessary to understand the underlying conflict that needs to be addressed. Having a positive attitude about finding a solution should motivate you into a productive conversation. Listen to the other person's concerns and ask for their solution to the problem. If the conversation develops into a blaming game or becomes heated, attempt to redirect the conversation into promoting a professional and fair solution. Partnering with a store manager or another pharmacist can be helpful to keep the conversation productive and assist in finding a solution.

For example, you are the new pharmacy manager and your lead technician Connie does not agree with your new policy to rotate workstations throughout the day. Connie states she refuses to move from her current workstation and undermines your authority as her supervisor. As the pharmacy manager, you should ask to speak with Connie outside of the pharmacy and ask why she is unwilling to move workstations. Connie states that she feels she is most proficient at data entry and complains that others make too many mistakes that she must go back and correct. Therefore, she would rather just do the work correctly herself. You should explain the need to allow others to improve as well as improve her skills in all aspects of the pharmacy to remain a top performer. Together, you can develop a plan for the pharmacy so other technicians can be aware of their mistakes and improve, while Connie assists in other workstations to improve her own skills.

If there is a conflict between two or more members of the support staff, the pharmacist is expected to listen to all sides individually and then bring all members together to determine a solution. If verbal conflict becomes a distraction to coworkers or customers, it is best to immediately escort the staff out of the pharmacy and call for store management to assist with the dispute. Once the situation has been defused, you will need to find the root cause of the escalation from each member. After listening to the individual sides, begin to anticipate challenges when the members come back

together to work on a solution so that you can redirect the conversation if it trends in a nonproductive direction. It is a best practice to have store management present for these discussions to provide insight and maintain composure of all parties.

For example, Kristin and Sarah are two technicians that have very different personalities. One day, Kristin snaps at Sarah when giving criticism to another technician and a verbal dispute takes place in the pharmacy. This disruption causes customers and other workers to become distracted by their conflict. At this point the pharmacist must remove the staff from the pharmacy and address the issues which have led up to this point. Kristin and Sarah should be separated to allow tensions to lower and regain composure to have a productive conversation. The pharmacist should listen to each side separately then ask Kristin and Sarah to come together to discuss their issues. Depending on the underlying issues, more coaching with each individual may be required to fully resolve the conflict between each party.

If there is a conflict between support staff and customers, immediately remove the staff member from the situation and take over. These conflicts are difficult because you may feel you are stuck between supporting your staff and ensuring the customer feels justified. If you uncover that the staff member is incorrect, then it is important to validate the staff member's intention to do the right thing when speaking to the customer. You may explain that they may have either had incorrect information or were unaware of specific details of this unique situation. If you uncover that the customer is incorrect, then calmly and thoroughly explain to the customer why the staff is correct, citing policy, law, or requirements. Some situations may continue to escalate and it would be appropriate to call for help from the store management or another pharmacist if available. If the conflict is over the phone, it is sometimes helpful to keep the customer on hold for a few seconds so that they can collect their thoughts and emotions before speaking with a supervisor. This can also give you a few moments to prepare yourself on how to defuse the situation. This can be accomplished by ensuring you listen to the issue or complaint, ask for their remedy to the situation, and be ready for some kind of solution.

For example, one of your customers, Mrs. Jones, is adamant that she does not need to provide her date of birth and address every time she comes to pick up a prescription and refuses to provide it to the cashier, in order to pick up her prescription. You are the pharmacist on duty, and you tell Mrs. Jones that because of the patient safety policy, the pharmacy requires this information every time a prescription is picked up. Mrs. Jones states she isn't consistently asked to, it is only with this particular cashier. You assure Mrs. Jones that the policy clearly states two patient identifiers must be checked with every sale of a prescription. It may be helpful to let Mrs. Jones know that you will retrain the staff so that the policy is followed consistently in the future.

If there is a conflict between two customers in the pharmacy area, immediately call for assistance by another staff member either in or out of the pharmacy department. As a pharmacist, it is your duty to keep the pharmacy secure and safe for everyone in the immediate vicinity, so do not engage or attempt to leave the pharmacy to resolve a conflict between customers.

For example, Mr. Brown is picking up his prescription at the pickup window while Mrs. Cline is waiting in line. Mrs. Cline's hands are full and she places her items on the pick-up counter while she waits her turn. Mr. Brown is offended that she is attempting to rush the transaction and asks her to step back. Mrs. Cline refuses to move. You, the pharmacist, kindly ask Mrs. Cline to wait further back in line due to HIPAA compliance, so that she cannot hear the conversation regarding Mr. Brown's transaction. At this point, Mr. Brown throws Mrs. Cline's items on the floor and continues with the transaction. You call the manager from the front store to assist with a customer in the pharmacy immediately, so he may assist with the conflict.

If a conflict is not resolved at the verbal level and results in physical contact, immediately ensure the safety of others and call for help from store management or police if needed. In no circumstance is physical contact acceptable and drastic measures should be avoided to ensure safety of yourself and your staff.

## ■ CONCLUSION

Many recent pharmacy graduates will find themselves in situations where they must exercise their human resources management skills, whether it is in the context of performance-related feedback, personal conflict, or workflow management. Unfortunately, pharmacy manager responsibilities such as recruitment and hiring and onboarding training is often taught on the job. Although companies have differing policies and situations have nuanced variability, the fundamental concepts introduced in this chapter help provide practical guidance for those with limited experience.

## ■ CHAPTER APPLICATIONS

1. You have an experienced technician that found a new employment opportunity and has decided to turn in her 2-week notice. Knowing that you will need to replace her in a timely manner, you need to create a job posting and description. What are the pharmacy technician qualifications that you need to include in the job posting?

2. Today is Wednesday at your pharmacy, and severe weather has reduced your sales for the week. You originally budgeted your schedule based on $89,500 of sales but now project you will only have $84,000 in sales.

   What is the amount of labor (in dollars) you budgeted for, based on 9.8% of sales? What is the new amount of labor (in dollars) you should project to use?

   Based on this difference, how would you cut labor hours to account for this loss in sales? Assume a technician at your pharmacy makes $15/h and a clerk makes $10/h.

3. As a new pharmacy manager, you have received several customer complaints that one of your pharmacists is rude to patients. You have not

worked overlapping shifts with this particular pharmacist for some time now, but it is your responsibility to address the issue. What is your approach to communicating this feedback to your pharmacist?

4. You are told by your lead technician that Carla, a technician, has been unusually rude and disrespectful to Betty, a cashier. Carla has been barking orders and not treating Betty with the same level of respect as the other staff members. How would you address this situation?

## REFERENCES

1. Shoemaker-Hunt S, McClellan S, Bacon O, et al. Cost of dispensing study. Abt Associates: Cambridge, MA, January 2020.
2. Dohrenwend, A. Serving up the feedback sandwich. *Fam Pract Manag.* 2002;9(10):43-46.
3. Goleman D, McKee A, Boyatzis RE. *Primal Leadership: Realizing the Power or Emotional Intelligence.* Boston, MA: Harvard Business School Press; 2002.

# 4

# OPTIMIZING PHARMACY WORKFLOW

*Mark Comfort, PharmD, and Nathan D. Pope, PharmD, BCACP, FACA*

---

## LEARNING OBJECTIVES

1. List the benefits of workflow optimization.
2. Identify ways to reduce waste and streamline workflow.
3. Describe how to improve efficiency and quality of the pharmacy workflow to improve patient satisfaction and grow profits.
4. Apply strategies to evaluate, organize, standardize, implement, and analyze pharmacy workflow for optimization.

## ■ SETTING THE SCENE

The contents of this chapter can be utilized and applied in all community pharmacy practice settings. Whether your practice site dispenses products, provides services, or does a combination of both, the ability to maintain and grow profits is necessary to run a successful business. Pharmacy, like many health care settings, is a competitive and quickly changing marketplace. You need to be able to adapt in order to stay relevant and to meet the needs of your customers. In this chapter, we will discuss ways to cut costs, save money, improve quality and safety, and ultimately provide better service to your customers. Accomplishing this will also free up your time in order to focus on growing other areas of your business. We understand that it may not be possible for you to implement all of the changes you would like to make. You may experience financial barriers, lack needed resources, such as technology, or you may not be the final decision maker in your organization. We recommend that you start with what you can control and implement those changes in your practice setting. Build from there. Sometimes even the smallest changes can have big impacts.

Imagine yourself in the following scenario: You have recently started as pharmacy manager for a community pharmacy that you have not worked at previously, and have been told by your boss that this pharmacy has many opportunities. Recently, there have been many customer complaints, some staff have either quit or transferred out to other pharmacies, and the overall financials of the pharmacy are not where they need to be. Your job is to improve customer satisfaction, employee satisfaction, and profitability of this pharmacy.

## ■ START WITH THE WHY

Before you design or implement anything, you need to understand the *Why*, *What*, and *How*.

- *Why*—Why are you doing this?
  - ○ Must align with your core values and the purpose that drives your organization[1]

- *What*—What are you promising?
  - ○ Defines the goal that you are promising to deliver
- *How*—How are you going to deliver?
  - ○ States the processes and procedures of how you will deliver on your promise

Additional questions that you can ask to help you identify the *Why*, *What*, and *How* are as follows.

### Why

1. Why are you considering this new change or process?
2. Why do you need this new change or process?
3. Does this new change or process align with your core values and/or mission statement?

### What

1. What is your goal?
2. What specifically do you want to accomplish?
3. What does success look like?

### How

1. How are you going to achieve this goal?
2. How specifically are you going to deliver?
3. How are you going to measure success?

Example: You own an independent pharmacy and your mission statement is: "We are the friendliest pharmacy in town … We know our customers by name and what they need."

Current problem: Your pharmacy is very busy. At times, the phone is constantly ringing, and there are not enough people working in the pharmacy to answer all of the lines. Customers or patients are waiting for long periods of time before someone helps them on the phone, resulting in dissatisfaction. In addition, the customers that are in the store are not getting helped as quickly as you would like because your employees are helping all of the customers on the phone.

To address this problem, you identify that WHAT you need is a way to reduce the number of phone calls in the pharmacy. You then decide HOW to do this by outsourcing some of your calls to a call center that is located in another town. This call center will now take most of your phone calls and allows your staff to have more time to help the customers in the pharmacy. It now appears that you have accomplished your goal. The new call center has improved your workflow efficiency and has led to better production and customer satisfaction.

However, you soon start receiving feedback from customers that every time they call they get somebody different on the phone. They say that the person on the phone tells them one thing, and then when they come to the pharmacy, they are told something different. You achieved your goal of decreasing phone calls into the pharmacy, but you have now created a new problem.

At this point, you start to ask yourself, "Why?" Why did I ever decide that the call center was the right thing to do? Why did I decide to utilize the call center in this manner? The problem here is that you did not start with the why. If you had, you may have decided that utilizing a call center in this manner never aligned with your pharmacy's mission statement of knowing your customers' names and needs.

Start with the WHY. Once you are satisfied with the WHY, you can move on to the WHAT and the HOW.

Your customer defines the value of the products or services you provide. Always try to view your business through the eyes of your customer. It may be efficient for you to outsource your phone calls; however, your customers also value the relationships they have developed with you and your staff. That relationship is a big part of what keeps them loyal to your business and you do not want to damage or lose that relationship. This does not mean that you should not utilize these types of resources. What it does mean is that you need to be mindful of HOW you implement them.

## ◼ IDENTIFY THE WHAT

Many health care settings today have, to some degree, implemented and benefited from techniques that are part of *Lean Six Sigma*.[2,3,4] Originally, these processes were developed for the managers of manufacturing plants. They combine the principles of Lean and Six

Sigma and have now expanded into other sectors of the economy including health care. The focus of Lean Six Sigma is to improve efficiency and quality by eliminating waste and reducing variation. We highly recommend that you further explore Lean Six Sigma as there are numerous texts available on this subject.

### Goal of Workflow Optimization

Improve processes → Improve Quality → Reduce Prices → Improve Customer Satisfaction → Increase Customer Loyalty → Grow Profits

### Evaluate

As you start at your new pharmacy, you may be tempted to implement changes right away. While this may be necessary in some areas, it is best to avoid making too many changes right away. Current staff are often nervous about change and are still getting to know you as a person and a manager. Initially, it is recommended to work on building relationships with your staff and patients. While you are doing this, you should be making observations and taking notes on how things currently operate and where the opportunities exist. Although you may have been told something in advance, it is always best to go in with a fresh set of eyes and make your own observations.

Ask your new staff how they feel the pharmacy is operating, what opportunities they feel exist, and what suggestions they have for improvement. Your staff may provide great input and suggestions, and you may be surprised at the solutions they come up with to address current issues. You don't have to take all of their suggestions, but it is important to engage staff and get their feedback throughout the process. You can also bounce ideas off of them by asking, "what do you think if we did this instead of that?" While some of your ideas may be excellent, it does not mean they will work for this specific pharmacy at this time.

As you go through this process you may hear your staff say, "We have always done it this way, so why do we need to do this differently now?" You may find it helpful to identify common ground with them. Find opportunities that you both agree upon and then work together to create solutions for them. Remember that just because it worked in the past does not mean it is going to work in the future. And it may not even work now!

As you are making your observations of current operations, here are some things to look for:

- *Bottlenecks*
  - Look for steps that are blocking the overall flow of the process. For instance, you find that your pharmacist is the bottleneck because they have too many tasks to complete. One solution would be to identify tasks that the pharmacist can delegate to others.
  - For example, pharmacy had the issue of a huge bottleneck at data entry. The data entry technician was constantly behind and customers were always upset because their prescription was not ready when promised. When the process was evaluated, it was discovered that management had not properly trained a clerk who was taking prescriptions at drop off. This clerk assumed everybody that dropped off a prescription was going to wait and needed the prescription as soon as possible. Because of this they were marking everything as urgent in the system and not properly prioritizing the work that needed to be completed. This was corrected by retraining the clerk to ask the patients, "when do you want to pick this up?" By correcting that one issue there was a dramatic improvement in workflow.
- *Waste*
  - This could be wasted time or waiting, overproduction, excess inventory, unnecessary or excessive motion, and even costly errors.
  - Extra-processing can also lead to waste if there are too many steps required to complete a task. Creating process flow maps can help you to streamline your workflow.
  - For example, another pharmacy had an issue with putting the order up each morning in a timely manner. When the process was observed, it was found that everyone utilized a different method, they touched each bottle more times than

necessary, and there was too much walking back and forth that took additional time. To address this issue, a new process was created and all staff were trained on the process. As they took the product out of the tote, they would place it into baskets that were labeled for different sections of the pharmacy (fast movers, refrigerator, over the counter, etc.). After organizing the order in baskets, they would take the baskets to those sections and place the products on the shelf where they belong. This new process significantly decreased the time it took to put up the order each day.

- *Staff productivity*
  - Look to see if you are utilizing your team to their full potential and getting them most out of their abilities. Identify which team members are the most productive and which are not in different roles in the pharmacy. Solutions to staff who are less productive may involve providing more training where it is needed. It can also involve providing adequate incentives to your team to help motivate and engage them.
  - Going back to the clerk mentioned earlier, he was known to have a bad attitude and was not an efficient worker. After observing this clerk for a couple of weeks, a few areas were identified that the clerk could be better utilized. This employee was retrained on the correct procedures for some processes and was also trained on how to complete additional tasks that they had not previously done. This employee's productivity level quickly increased and they became more engaged and satisfied with their role on the team.

## ■ WORK ON THE HOW

### Organize

Sort and Remove → Set Locations → Systematize

Once you have identified areas of waste or processes that need improvement, it is time to organize. Organization is an important part of improving workflow efficiency. An organized workspace will help you to increase productivity by saving time, reducing stress, and allowing you time to focus on the task at hand. The goal is to be able to find what you need, when you need it, without wasting time.

Start by removing all unnecessary equipment or clutter that you do not need. A good way to do this is to create three separate baskets:

- Basket #1: Items you know you want to keep
- Basket #2: Items you don't need and can get rid of
- Basket #3: Items that you are not sure about

Once you get rid of the items in basket #2, you will already feel a big sense of accomplishment. It is recommended to keep the items in basket #3 for only a short time. If after a week or two you still haven't taken an item out of basket #3, then you probably don't need it and can discard it. Take advantage of your de-cluttered workspace and give everything a good cleaning. You might be surprised to see how much dust and dirt you find!

After you are done removing unnecessary clutter and cleaning up, it is time to set locations for the items you want to keep. For each area of your pharmacy, determine the items you use most often for tasks that you complete in each designated area. Make a list of these items as you go. You will want these items close to you so that they are easy to find when you need them. If it is something that you use multiple times an hour, then you will want that item within arm's reach. For items that you use less frequently, it is okay to place them a little further away, such as, under the counter or in a drawer. Put some thought into where you want items to be located in order to be the most productive. Pick locations that make sense and are convenient for you and others on your team.

As you set locations for items, it is helpful to add labels where appropriate. Label the outside of a drawer or cabinet so everyone will know what is in it. Label the areas inside the drawer or cabinet so everyone will know where to put the items that go inside. By doing this you will create a home for all of the important items in your pharmacy. If you don't label items and their locations, then you may find that over time they will tend to "walk off" and disappear. At one

pharmacy there was a problem finding staplers and scissors. These items would always wander off, and it always took extra time to find them when you needed it. To address this, more of these items were purchased and placed in all the locations in the pharmacy that needed them. Then they were all labeled so everyone would know which area they belonged, just in case they tried to wander off again!

Don't let all of this hard work go to waste. Create a process to maintain the cleanliness and organization of your pharmacy. A great way to do this is to create checklists. A daily checklist can be utilized for basic cleaning and to make sure items return to their home locations at the end of the day. Weekly or monthly checklists can be utilized for deep cleaning and reorganization as needed (see Figure 4-1 for an example of checklist). You can use the lists of items you created for each area to create visual training aids to help reinforce what does and does not belong in each area for all pharmacy personnel.

## Standardize

Now that you have a leaner, cleaner, and more organized pharmacy, you need to create standardized workflow processes and procedures for your pharmacy personnel to utilize. Standardization eliminates guesswork by clearly defining what tasks need to be completed and how they will be done. If all staff members follow these standardized processes, there will be quality improvement in workflow, productivity, and job satisfaction.

Standardization promotes all team members completing tasks in the same manner and hopefully with the same level of efficiency. If you have multiple pharmacy locations, standardization will guarantee that productivity and quality are the same across all locations. Small improvements can have big impacts, especially if they involve tasks that are repeated regularly. Improvements can have exponential impacts if they are implemented at multiple pharmacy locations.

First, you will need to identify what the optimal process or procedure looks like for your pharmacy. You may need to invest further time and resources into

---

**Pharmacy Organization Checklist**

☐ **Daily**
    ☐ Return drugs to shelf
    ☐ Restock supplies (lids, vials, bags, etc.)
    ☐ Return items to home locations
    ☐ Clean
        ☐ Counter surfaces
        ☐ Counting trays and machines
        ☐ Sink
    ☐ Remove boxes or other items from the floor
    ☐ Empty trash and throw away boxes

☐ **Weekly**
    ☐ Wipe down items and equipment on top of counter
    ☐ Clean floors and mats in entire pharmacy
    ☐ Reorder supplies
    ☐ Remove and replace signage as needed

☐ **Monthly**
    ☐ All items have a home location and are labeled (Reorganize as needed)
    ☐ Remove any unused items (Keep in the holding area for no more than 1 month)
    ☐ Discard items in holding area if no longer needed.
    ☐ Deep clean pharmacy
        ☐ Areas under counters
        ☐ Shelves
        ☐ Vents, air filters, sprinkler system
        ☐ Items outside of pharmacy
            ☐ Line ropes
            ☐ Sign holders
            ☐ Blood pressure machine
            ☐ Outside walls of pharmacy
    ☐ Update this checklist if needed

**Figure 4-1.** Pharmacy organization checklist example.

studying these processes and procedures to look for opportunities for improvement. Sometimes you may have to try different approaches until you learn which one works the best. Again, work with your staff and get their ideas and suggestions throughout the process. You need their input and will want their buy-in for the best chance of success.

Once you have identified what the optimal process or procedure looks like, you will need to create *standard operating procedures (SOPs)*. Start with the processes and procedures you identified as opportunities during the evaluation phase. These SOPs need to detail specifically what needs to be done, how it is done, who does it, and how they do it. SOPs help

all staff better understand their roles, what tasks they need to complete, and how to complete them. Eventually you will want to create SOPs for all major workstations or tasks that are completed in the pharmacy. These SOPs should be reviewed and updated at least annually.

## Implement

Create a plan in advance on how you will implement this new SOP. This plan should include the resources needed and a timeline for SOP implementation. Involve the leaders and key members of your team with developing this plan. Their input and support are key ingredients to successful implementation.

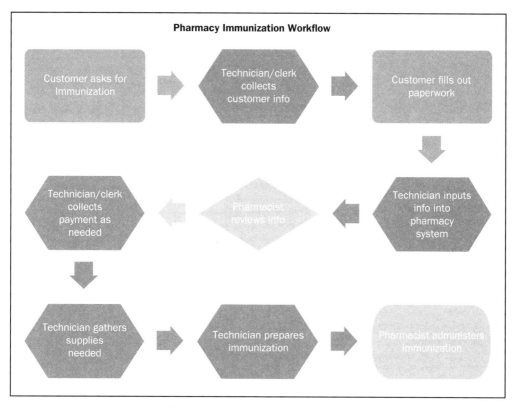

**Figure 4-2.** Process flowchart example.

They can also be utilized as champions to help lead your team throughout this change. Before you initiate the new process or procedure, you need to clearly communicate the *Why*, *What*, and *How* to your team.

- *Why*: They need to understand why this is needed in order to obtain buy-in. Tell them how this will benefit them, the business, and your customers.
- *What*: Define the goal and explain to your team what success looks like.
- *How*: Share the new SOP with them. Make sure they understand how the process or procedure should be completed going forward.

Make sure your team knows that you support this change. Your team will watch what you do, and it is critical that you lead by example. They will follow your actions more than your words so you need to make sure you are doing what you are asking them to do. Get commitments from your team. Ask them to commit to giving this new process a try and to give you feedback throughout the change. Let them know that their feedback is important and will be used to help revise and improve the process.

Time needs to be allocated to train your team. They will need instruction at the beginning and coaching throughout to ensure competency and efficiency. Praise them when they are doing things correctly, and this will provide positive reinforcement. Feedback should also be given when appropriate to ensure that the new SOP is being followed. Process flowcharts can be created and utilized as teaching tools and resources (see Figure 4-2 for an example of Process Flowchart). They should detail each step in the process from start to finish. *Visual training aids* can be created and placed in logical locations to help reinforce the steps in the process.

## Analyze

You now need to evaluate the results to determine if you have achieved your goal or if improvements need to be made. One of the best ways to analyze productivity is by measuring it. This can not only help you determine if the overall process has improved, but it can also help you determine how various steps in the process have changed. Another way to measure success is by getting feedback from your customers and staff. Ask your customers if they are seeing a difference in your operations. Ask your staff if this new process is helping them or making their job duties easier to perform. Whenever possible, collect data and share this with your team. They may be surprised to see what the data says, and this can help them to better understand the benefits of the new process.

Be ready to make adjustments to the process as needed. Analyze what is working and what is not. If improvements are needed, you can update your process and evaluate further. It is recommended to only make one or two adjustments at a time. If you make too many adjustments, then it is difficult to determine the effect of each. Continuing to analyze and adjust your process is known as *continuous quality improvement (CQI)*. CQI is an ongoing process that you can utilize to optimize your pharmacy workflow.

## Additional Considerations: Automation

Automation and enhancements in technology can also have big impacts. They can help improve productivity and can also improve your overall customer experience. Automated counting devices, dispensing systems, inventory systems, ordering systems, etc., can not only save your pharmacy time but can also reduce human error and improve quality. Enhancements in technology can be utilized to improve the efficiency of your operating system, customer interface, documentation system, records management, training,

communication, etc. When possible it is highly recommended to consider automation and technology enhancements as part of your CQI process.

## ■ CHAPTER APPLICATIONS

Complete the following worksheet to implement workflow improvements in your pharmacy where you are working or are on rotation.

Step 1: Identify 3–4 areas of your pharmacy workflow that you would like to improve:

_____

Step 2: From this list, select one area where improvement is most needed and that will increase your bottom-line profits.

_____

Step 3: For the area of improvement selected, identify:

- *Why*: Why are you doing this? _____
- *What*: What are you promising? _____
- *How*: How are you going to deliver?
  - What needs to be done? _____
  - How is it done? _____
  - Who does what? _____
  - How do they do it? _____

## REFERENCES

1. Sinek S. *Start with Why: How Great Leaders Inspire Everyone to Take Action*. London: Portfolio Penguin; 2011.
2. George ML. *Lean Six Sigma: Combining Six Sigma Quality with Lean Speed*. New York, NY: McGraw-Hill; 2002.
3. George ML, Rowlands D, Kastle B. *What Is Lean Six Sigma?* New York, NY: McGraw-Hill; 2004.
4. Lean Six Sigma in the Pharmacy Department. pharmacytimes.com. Published September 17, 2019. Accessed January 24, 2021. https://www.pharmacytimes.com/publications/health-system-edition/2014/september2014/lean-six-sigma-in-the-pharmacy-department

# 5

# COMMON LEGAL ASPECTS OF PHARMACY PRACTICE

*Rachel E. Barenie, PharmD, JD, MPH, Carol A. Schwab, JD, LLM, and Tyler Dinkelaker, PharmD, JD, MBA*

---

### ▨ LEARNING OBJECTIVES

1. Identify controlled substance prescriptions that are not issued for a legitimate medical purpose.
2. Recall key HIPAA-related concepts and describe common compliance issues.
3. Describe three federal statutes used to prohibit and enforce health-care fraud.
4. Identify resources to remain up-to-date on state and federal pharmacy law changes.

Pharmacy practice is ever-evolving, and the same can be said for the laws and regulations that govern it. Even though states are the primary regulators of pharmacy practice, many governmental entities influence—both directly and indirectly—the daily operations and decisions that must be made to provide high quality patient care. Always remember, the rules and regulations serve as a framework for which pharmacists must practice within, but they alone are not enough to ensure competence. We encourage you to use the laws and regulations as another tool in your best-practices toolkit to serve your patients, knowing that it will likely raise more questions than it answers. This chapter cannot possibly reteach you pharmacy law, especially considering the substantial variation that exists among states. Instead, this chapter is structured to discuss key issues that community pharmacists encounter every day in practice—controlled substances, HIPAA, healthcare fraud, and tips for staying up-to-date.

Disclaimer: The readers must note that this chapter is for educational purposes only and is not intended to represent legal advice. If you have specific legal questions, please consult an attorney.

# ■ CONTROLLED SUBSTANCES

While controlled substances represent a small portion of all prescription drugs, they are the most highly regulated. Pharmacists are at the greatest risk of losing their license or being criminally charged with illegal drug diversion when these regulations are not followed. An excellent overview of these rules is the manual of the Drug Enforcement Agency (DEA) manual for pharmacists,[1] and community pharmacists should be familiar with this manual.

Prescriptions for controlled substances must be for a legitimate medical purpose issued by an individual practitioner acting in the usual course of his or her professional practice.[2] Although the prescriber has the primary responsibility to ensure the legitimacy of controlled substance prescriptions, pharmacists have a corresponding responsibility to dispense controlled substances only for legitimate medical purposes.[2] If the pharmacist knew, or should have known, that a prescription was not issued for a legitimate medical purpose, the pharmacist may be held civilly and criminally liable.[3] Because of the potential serious consequences to both pharmacists and patients, pharmacists must be able to identify prescriptions that are illegal on their face, and to identify red flags that indicate a prescription is not for a legitimate medical purpose.[4] Here are a few examples of prescriptions that should raise red flags for community pharmacists.

*Scenario #1. A patient presents a prescription for oxycodone 5 mg #15 for a 7-day supply to be taken as needed for extreme low back pain that was issued 8 months ago.* Federal regulations do not put an expiration date on Schedule II prescriptions (unlike the 6-month expiration date on Schedule III and IV drugs). State law may indicate an expiration date for Schedule II prescriptions, ranging from 30 days to a year. In this scenario, the pharmacist must determine whether the medication is still for a legitimate medical purpose, especially since it was issued for acute use and the patient has not needed the medication for 8 months.[1]

*Scenario #2. A pediatrician issues a prescription for oxycodone to a patient's parent for severe pain.* This prescription is illegal if it is outside the prescribing authority of the prescriber, or if it is not written for a legitimate medical purpose. A pediatrician is either an M.D. or a D.O, who has full prescribing authority which is determined by state law and professional licensing boards.[5] The prescribing authority for physicians is determined by their license to practice medicine and surgery—not by their subspecialty certification. A pediatrician is not limited to writing prescriptions for children. The appropriate inquiry is whether the prescription was written for a legitimate medical purpose, and pain is a legitimate medical purpose. Other professionals with prescribing authority, such as dentists, are limited to prescribing for purposes related to their area of licensure—dentistry. Mid-level practitioners, such as nurse practitioners or physician assistants, are limited by the protocols established with their collaborating or supervising physicians.[5]

*Scenario #3. An individual practitioner issues a prescription for "office stock" of a controlled substance for patients undergoing in-office procedures.* This prescription is illegal on its face.[2] Prescriptions for controlled substances should be written for identified patients.

*Scenario #4. A physician calls in a prescription for oxycodone and tells the pharmacist it is an emergency for a patient who is in a lot of pain due to a fall.* The issue is whether this scenario meets the definition of "emergency" that justifies an oral Schedule II prescription. Federal regulations define "emergency" to mean that immediate administration of the controlled substance is necessary for the proper treatment of the patient; no appropriate alternative treatment is available; and it is not reasonably possible for the prescribing physician to provide a written prescription to the pharmacist before dispensing.[6] If there are alternatives that can effectively manage the patient's pain, it is not an emergency, and the oral Schedule II prescription would be illegal.

*Scenario #5. A patient presents three separate prescriptions for oxycodone, each for a 30-day supply. One is dated for today's date, June 1, the second is dated for July 1, and the third is dated for July 31.* The only prescription that may be dispensed is the prescription dated for June 1. The other two prescriptions are post-dated and are illegal under federal regulations, which require that all prescriptions for controlled substances be dated and signed on the date issued.[7] The appropriate format would be to date all three of the prescriptions for the date they were issued with instructions indicating the earliest date each prescription may be dispensed.

*Scenario #6. On August 5, a patient presents a prescription for a 30-day supply of oxycodone and requests that the prescription be dispensed 10 tablets at a time to help the patient afford the medication. The prescription was issued on August 1.* Federal law permits this transaction if the following requirements are met: the transaction is consistent with state law, the total amount dispensed does not exceed a 30-day supply, and all dispensing occurs within 30 days after the prescription was issued.[8] The last day that the pharmacist may dispense a partial fill is August 31. If state law does not permit a partial fill over a 30-day period, the balance of the prescription must be ready for dispensing within 72 hours of the first partial filling. However, the DEA takes the position that the patient does not need to pick up the prescription within that 72-hour limit.[1]

*Scenario #7. A patient presents a prescription for methadone, and the pharmacist knows that this patient is being treated for opioid use disorder (OUD).* This is an illegal prescription because methadone may not be prescribed to treat OUD in the general course of practicing medicine.[9] While methadone is approved by the Food and Drug Administration (FDA) to treat OUD, that treatment can only be provided through certified opioid treatment programs that are registered with the DEA. Within these treatment programs, methadone may be dispensed or administered, but not prescribed,[10] so a community pharmacist should not see a prescription written for methadone for the treatment of OUD. The only prescriptions a community pharmacist should see for OUD are prescriptions written for FDA-approved buprenorphine products by a qualifying practitioner who has (or who has applied for) a Drug Addiction Treatment Act waiver number ("X waiver").[11]

These scenarios represent only a few examples of the legal issues that may arise in dispensing controlled substances. Each pharmacist must use his or her professional judgment in determining the best course of action when confronted with a prescription that raises a red flag.

## ◼ HIPAA HIGHLIGHTS

HIPAA, a federal law with the formal title of the Health Insurance Portability and Accountability Act of 1996, balances protecting an individual's identifying information with promoting the continuity of high quality healthcare and the public health at-large.[12] Most often in healthcare the question is not "what is HIPAA?"

but rather "how does someone comply with HIPAA?" This question becomes increasingly important as new health-related technologies are developed, health information and data are shared more easily and seamlessly, and connecting with patients, providers, insurers, and others virtually becomes the new norm.

Understanding "who" HIPAA applies to and "what" HIPAA requires is the first step in complying with this law. A *covered entity* is the "who," such as a community pharmacist treating individuals (i.e., patients!). *Business associates* of covered entities are also required to comply.[13,14,15] The "what" is *protected health information (PHI)*, or simply any health information that can identify an individual, such as name, picture, email, or prescription number, as examples seen in Table 5-1.[14] HIPAA requires a covered entity not to use or disclose PHI, unless *required* or *permitted* by law or *authorized* by the individual in writing.[16]

There are instances when disclosure of PHI is required, including when an individual requests access to their PHI and when required by the Department of Health and Human Services[16] or by state law (i.e., reporting child abuse or communicable disease). There are many instances where permitted disclosures are allowed, and the decision to disclose rests with the professional judgment of the covered entity (e.g., you, the pharmacist!).[16] If the disclosure is not required or permitted by law, it must be authorized by the individual in writing.[17] Except under very limited circumstances, providing care to individuals cannot be conditioned on patient authorization for use or disclosure.[17] Remember, *de-identified* health information (i.e., all identifying information is removed) is not PHI, and therefore not protected under HIPAA.[16,18]

## Prescription Drug Monitoring … Problems

In 2019, Board of Pharmacy investigators found that a pharmacist accessed the state's prescription drug monitoring database 39 times for persons that were not patients. The Board revoked his license and referred the HIPAA incident to the Office of Civil Rights (OCR).[19]

When using or disclosing PHI, the *minimum necessary standard* often applies, meaning you should only use or disclose as little information as possible to provide the necessary care.[16,18] This principle always applies to sharing PHI with business associates, and pharmacies must have business associate agreements in place before sharing any PHI.[16] The minimum necessary standard does not apply for treatment purposes.[16]

All covered entities are required to develop and implement a *notice of privacy practice (NPP)* and policies and procedures ensuring compliance with HIPAA. The HIPAA NPP must be posted in the pharmacy and online, if the pharmacy maintains a website.[20] When a direct treatment relationship exists, such as between a pharmacist and patient, the patient must be provided notice of the pharmacy's HIPAA NPP during the first visit that services are provided, and the pharmacy must make a good faith effort to obtain a written acknowledgment each individual received the notice.

### We Need a Policy for That?

In 2009, a nationally known pharmacy chain paid $2.25 million in part because they did not have proper policies and procedures in place to safeguard PHI and failed to provide adequate training on those policies![21]

Just as notice is necessary, so are proper safeguards and disposal procedures for PHI. For example, covered entities must implement reasonable and appropriate safeguards to ensure confidentiality (i.e., not available or disclosed to unauthorized persons) and thwart threats.[22] PHI must always be protected and disposed of, including electronic media, properly. Moreover, an entity's team must be trained on these procedures, including volunteers.[20]

### A Very Expensive Laptop

In 2017, a hospital employee's unencrypted laptop containing PHI of about 20 431 individuals was stolen. Upon further investigation, the OCR found the organization did not comply with their own policies that indicated laptops and other devices be encrypted. The organization paid over $1 million for this breach.[23]

### From Trash to … Trouble!

In 2010, a nationally known pharmacy chain paid $1 million for not properly disposing of PHI. The chain

**Table 5-1. HIPAA Highlights**

| Key concept | | Notes/Examples |
|---|---|---|
| Who must comply with HIPAA? | • Covered entities<br>• Business associates of covered entities | Covered entities:<br>• Health plans<br>• Healthcare clearinghouses<br>• Healthcare providers, including individuals, who transmit any health information in electronic form for financial and administrative purposes (billing, payment, coverage status, and others) |
| Who is a business associate? | Person or organization that performs functions for or provides services to the covered entity that involves the use or disclosure of PHI. | A business associate is not an employee of the covered entity. Functions performed may include claims processing, utilization review, or billing, and more. Services provided are more limited and include legal, actuarial, accounting, consulting, data aggregation, management, administrative, accreditation, or financial services. |
| What is PHI? | Individually identifiable health information held or transmitted by a covered entity or its business associate | • May be in any form or media (electronic, paper, or oral)<br>• May be related to individual's past, present, or future care, or any payment for or provision of that care, that could reasonably be used to identify the individual |
| What is de-identified health information? | Health information that does not identify an individual and there is no reasonable basis to believe that it could be used to identify an individual. | Possible identifiers: Name; address; all elements of data (except year) that directly relate to an individual; telephone number; fax number; email; social security number; health plan beneficiary number; account number; vehicle identifiers; device identifies; URLs; IP address; biometric identifies (finger and voice prints); full face photos and any comparable images; and any other unique identifying number, characteristic, or code |
| What are lawful uses and disclosures of PHI? | • Required uses and disclosures | • Individuals (or their personal representatives) who request access to their PHI and/or an accounting of past PHI disclosures<br>• As required by the Department of Health and Human Services for compliance, investigative, or enforcement purposes<br>• As required by state law |

*(Continued)*

**Table 5-1. HIPAA Highlights (*Continued*)**

| Key concept | Notes/Examples |
|---|---|
| • Permitted uses and disclosures | • To the individual (who is the subject of the information) or to a personal representative of the individual<br>• For treatment (e.g., prior authorizations, refill reminders, dispensing, counseling), payment (e.g., submitting insurance claims, determining insurance coverage/eligibility), or healthcare operations (e.g., quality assessment, performance reviews, fraud detection, audits, business management)<br>• When the individual has the opportunity to agree or object to the use or disclosure (e.g., when the individual is asked outright)<br>• Incidental (occurs as a result of) to an otherwise permitted use, so long as reasonable safeguards are in place and minimum necessary principle applied<br>• Limited data set<br>• Public interest and benefit activities:<br>  ○ Required by law (reporting to the prescription drug monitoring program)<br>  ○ Victims of abuse, neglect, or domestic violence<br>  ○ Health oversight activities<br>  ○ Judicial and administrative proceedings<br>  ○ Law enforcement purposes<br>  ○ Public health activities<br>  ○ Decedents<br>  ○ Cadaveric organ, eye, or tissue donation<br>  ○ Research<br>  ○ Serious threats to health and safety<br>  ○ Essential government functions<br>  ○ Worker's compensation |
| • Authorized uses and disclosures (patient authorization obtained) | • Psychotherapy notes, unless an exception applies<br>• Marketing<br>• Sale |

HIPAA, Health Insurance Portability and Accountability Act of 1996; PHI, protected health information

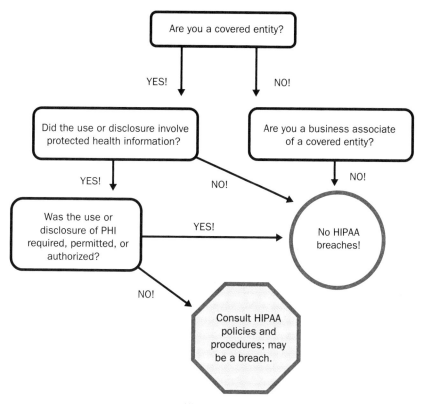

**Figure 5-1.** HIPAA breach flowchart.

disposed of used, and still labeled, prescription bottles in their industrial trash bin that was accessible by the general public.[21,24]

Without adequate policies and procedures in place, a breach of HIPAA could occur. A HIPAA breach generally occurs when PHI is accessed, used, or disclosed in an unpermitted way that compromises its security or privacy (Figure 5-1).[25] Breaches can be costly—to both the pharmacy and the individual. The top three most common compliance issues, as reported by OCR, are: impermissible uses and disclosures of PHI; lack of PHI safeguards; and lack of patient access to their own PHI.[26] Knowing your organization's HIPAA policies and procedures is critical to complying with HIPAA (i.e., avoiding a breach) and mitigating the disastrous effects if one occurs. To sum up this section on HIPAA: when in doubt, don't give that PHI out!

## ■ HEALTHCARE FRAUD

Hopefully a pharmacist will never experience a healthcare fraud situation in their pharmacy career, but it can be more common than one thinks. There are many types of healthcare fraud, and this brief overview is intended to serve as a starting point to help pharmacists understand and avoid improper transactions and relationships that may lead to claims of fraud in the pharmacy.

### Federal False Claims Act

At its simplest, the *Federal False Claims Act (FCA)* makes it illegal for anyone to submit, or cause submission, of a false or fraudulent claim to the government for payment.[27] In healthcare, Medicare or Medicaid are two of the most obvious government payers that pharmacies frequently submit claims for reimbursement. The FCA also requires that an individual act knowingly.[28] However, acting with deliberate ignorance or reckless disregard to the truth may also satisfy the intent needed under the FCA.[29]

Examining an FCA violation from a case in California helps put a pharmacist's action into context when considering what is a "false claim." In this case, the pharmacist-owner was found guilty of carrying out a scheme to submit claim information for prescriptions that were not dispensed or picked up.[30] The owner knowingly submitted these claims to Medicare and subsequently plead guilty and served 18 months in federal prison.[30]

False claims can include other improper billing practices like up-coding and submitting undocumented or untruthful claims.[31] For example, reusing nursing-home medications from other patients without crediting the previous patient's account,[32] billing claims for deceased patients, or overbilling a service or medication could all be considered false claims.

Penalties for false claims can be up to 3 times the amount of the claim submitted plus additional civil monetary penalties.[28] Moreover, a provider may also be excluded from participating in federal healthcare plans.

## Federal Anti-Kickback Statute

Anti-Kickback Statute (AKS) prevents an individual from knowingly soliciting or offering *remuneration* in exchange for a good or service that will be paid in full or part by federal healthcare programs.[33] Here is an example:

John Doe, a pharmacist, needs business. John tells his friend, a local doctor (practicing geriatric rheumatology), he'll pay the doctor $50 cash for each of the practice's patients that fill a compounded pain cream at John's pharmacy.

Here, John (anyone), knowingly offers $50 (remuneration), in exchange for a referral (the prescription

for compounded pain cream). This meets the first parts of an AKS violation, but the last component—paid in full or part by a federal healthcare program—is unknown. Since the doctor specializes in geriatrics (eligible for Medicare), it can be assumed that at least some of the claims would meet the last component regarding payment of the claim. Even if no claims are paid by the federal government, John may still be violating state law, or even provisions of his insurance contracts.

It is important to note that AKS has many exceptions (i.e., "safe harbors") that include referral services, coupons, warranties, discounts and group purchasing organizations, employees, and personal service and management contracts.[34] *Safe harbors* are detailed, can be extremely complicated, and often have many requirements to satisfy to eliminate any potential liability under the law. For other examples, please visit the Department of Justice's website and view the press releases and enforcement actions.[35]

## Physician Self-Referral: Stark Law

Understanding prohibitions of physician self-referral (Stark Law) is important because the law is free of any requisite intent. Therefore, one could be guilty of a Stark Law violation, even if they didn't know they were violating the law!

So, what is the Stark Law? Stark Law makes it unlawful for a physician or immediate family member(s) to financially gain from a referral for designated health services to an entity that is paid in whole or part for these services by a government payer.[36] Sound familiar? It should! The Stark Law, however, specifically involves a physician or their immediate family member(s) who benefits from the referral.

An example of a potential Stark Law violation would include a local physician investing in the town's pharmacy and then referring patients to that pharmacy. Stark Law can also be implicated when pharmacies or drug companies exceed specific limits of non-cash gratuities (meals, entertainment, conference registration, etc.).[37] Penalties for violations of Stark Law include civil monetary fines and possible exclusion from participation in federal programs.[38] There are many more examples of Stark Law violations, but remember, to be differentiated from AKS, the violation must include a physician or their immediate family member.

## Whistleblower Actions

A *qui tam* action is a whistleblower lawsuit filed by a private individual, known as a relator, on behalf of the government when fraud is suspected. Sometimes the government steps in to take over the action; if the government prevails, the individual could receive between 15 and 30% of the money recovered. *Qui tam* actions make a large part of the government's enforcement actions, and in 2019, over $2.1 billion was recovered because of these filed actions enforcing the statutes previously mentioned.[39]

Healthcare fraud is ever present within the U.S. healthcare system and continues to risk patient care and trust in the pharmacy profession. It is a pharmacist's job to engage in legal and ethical behavior at all times and to avoid even the perception of fraudulent activity.

## ■ TIPS FOR STAYING UP-TO-DATE

We highlighted a few notable areas of federal law that have shaped how pharmacy is practiced today. However, pharmacy practice is ever changing and affected by many rules and regulations so it's imperative that you stay up-to-date. Remember, it is your license and responsibility to practice within the framework the law allows. So how do you do this?

### #1 Use Reputable and Reliable Sources

Pharmacists should seek reputable and reliable sources for their pharmacy law information. These resources include government agencies (e.g., Drug Enforcement Agency, Food and Drug Administration), regulatory boards (e.g., state Boards of Pharmacy, Departments of Health), and national and state pharmacy associations. For example, some of these organizations publish quarterly newsletters highlighting important updates and a Board's current thinking on a topic or issue. Another opportunity is attending law-focused continuing education, which may or not already be required in your state. This information can be tremendously helpful as it is state-specific and contains a manageable amount of information.

### #2 Review Sources Regularly

Pharmacists should review their resources often. Laws and regulations are constantly evolving as regulatory bodies catch up to concerns or advances in pharmacy and healthcare. Moreover, most state legislatures pass legislation impacting your practice each year, so reviewing these updates from reputable sources regularly is important.

### #3 Know How a Change Impacts Your Practice, if at All

When identifying a change relevant to your practice, it is important to understand what that change means. The law can be very complex and sometimes difficult to interpret. Thus, it is important to remember that the Board is a resource to provide insight. For example, if a question arises where the answer is not clear or you are unsure how a new change to the law or Board rules will impact your day-to-day practice, a good next step may be reaching out to the Board for help.

## ■ CONCLUSION

This chapter briefly summarizes only a few common issues pharmacists practicing in community pharmacy may encounter daily. It is imperative that pharmacists not only know and understand the law, but also stay up-to-date with rapidly changing rules and regulations. At the end of the day, it is the pharmacist's licensure and, thus, the pharmacist's responsibility to practice within the bounds of the law.

## ■ CHAPTER APPLICATIONS

1. A pharmacist receives a prescription from John Smith, DDS for hydrocodone and acetaminophen. In conformance with state law, Dr. Smith included the ICD-10 diagnostic code on the prescription order. The pharmacist looks up the meaning of the code online and learns that the patient is being treated for back pain.

2. On a Friday evening an hour before closing, a pharmacist receives a call from a physician who wants to orally issue a prescription order for oxycodone hydrochloride extended-release tablets. The prescription order is for a cancer patient in a nursing home, and the nurse administered the patient's last tablet earlier that evening. Other pain medications have been tried for this patient, but none have been as effective as this medication. The physician is out of town for the weekend on a camping trip and will be unable to issue a written prescription order, either in hard copy or electronically, until Monday morning.[6,40]

3. Patient reports filling medications at multiple pharmacies in her community to obtain the lowest prescription drug price. The patient explains that she is trying to identify an insurance plan that will help her lower her prescription costs and requests a copy of all prescriptions filled in the last year at your pharmacy.[41]

4. A Board of Pharmacy inspector visits your pharmacy based on reports that a prescriber in your community is writing prescriptions in violation of state law. The inspector requests all prescriptions written by that prescriber and dispensed at your pharmacy be made available for inspection.[42]

5. A local physician invites you, the town's only pharmacy owner, to dinner one evening and proposes that you should open a medical equipment and supply store. There is no other store in town and the aging population in your small rural town could surely benefit from having access to much needed medical equipment. Moreover, you are an expert when it comes to medical billing and the physician uses an outside service. The physician proposes to be your silent partner with seed money and only asks for a small percentage of the profits in return. If everything was agreeable to you, the physician would send over the paperwork in the morning from his attorney. Do you sign the papers? Why or why not?

6. The pharmacy's new marketing manager comes to you with several ideas about new promotions and ways to drive customers in the door. One idea the manager proposes is to start a rewards club where the pharmacy waives up to 3 generic medication copays a month—no-questions asked. He thinks that since the generics don't cost that much and that copays are generally low, the plan could really get people in the door to buy other items and wants to know what you think?

## REFERENCES

1. Drug Enforcement Agency. Pharmacist's Manual: An Informational Outline of the Controlled Substances Act. Revised 2020. Washington, DC: DEA; 2020. Accessed May 21, 2021. https://www.deadiversion.usdoj.gov/GDP/(DEA-DC-046)(EO-DEA154)_Pharmacist_Manual.pdf
2. 21 CFR §1306.04.
3. *United States v Lawson*, 682 F2d 480 (4th Cir 1982).
4. The National Association of Boards of Pharmacy® (NABP®) and the Anti-Diversion Industry Working Group (ADIWG), a consortium of pharmaceutical manufacturers and distributors, created an educational video for pharmacists to help them identify the warning signs of prescription drug abuse and diversion when dispensing controlled substance prescriptions. The video, entitled, "Red Flags," was released at the NABP 110th Annual Meeting. Accessed May 21, 2021. https://www.youtube.com/watch?v=WY9BDgcdxaM
5. 21 CFR §1306.03.
6. 21 CFR §290.10.
7. 21 CFR §1306.05, 21 CFR §1306.12.

8. 21 USC §829; 21 CFR §1306.13.

9. 21 CFR §1306.04(c); 21 CFR §1306.07.

10. 21 CFR §1306.07.

11. 21 CFR §1301.28.

12. Public Law No. 104-191, 110 Stat 1936 (1996).

13. 45 CFR §160.102.

14. 45 CFR §160.103.

15. Centers for Medicare and Medicaid Services (CMS). Covered Entity guidance. Baltimore, MD: CMS; 2020. Accessed May 21, 2021. https://www.cms.gov/Regulations-and-Guidance/Administrative-Simplification/HIPAA-ACA/Downloads/CoveredEntitiesChart20160617.pdf

16. 45 CFR §164.502.

17. 45 CFR §164.501.

18. 45 CFR §164.514.

19. Tennessee Board of Pharmacy. Board Meeting Minutes, November 5–6, 2020. Nashville, TN: Tennessee State Government; 2019. Accessed May 21, 2021. https://www.tn.gov/content/dam/tn/health/healthprofboards/pharmacy/Mins11-19.pdf

20. 45 CFR §164.530.

21. Department of Health and Human Services (HHS). Resolution Agreement: CVS Pays $2.5 Million & Toughens Disposal Practices to Settle HIPAA Privacy Case. Washington, DC: HHS; 2017. Accessed May 21, 2021. https://www.hhs.gov/hipaa/for-professionals/compliance-enforcement/examples/cvs/index.html

22. 45 CFR §164.306.

23. Lifespan pays $1,040,000 to OCR to settle unencrypted stolen laptop breach. Department of Health and Human Services (HHS). 2020. Accessed May 21, 2021. https://www.hhs.gov/about/news/2020/07/27/lifespan-pays-1040000-ocr-settle-unencrypted-stolen-laptop-breach.html

24. Department of Health and Human Services (HHS). Rite Aid Agrees to pay $1 Million to Settle HIPAA Privacy Case. Washington, DC: HHS; 2017. Accessed May 21, 2021. https://www.hhs.gov/hipaa/for-professionals/compliance-enforcement/examples/rite-aid/index.html

25. 45 CFR §164.400.

26. Department of Health and Human Services (HHS). Enforcement Highlights. Washington, DC: HHS; 2020. Accessed May 21, 2021. https://www.hhs.gov/hipaa/for-professionals/compliance-enforcement/data/enforcement-highlights/index.html

27. 31 USC §3729(a).

28. 31 USC §3729(a)(1).

29. 31 USC §3729(b)(1).

30. Department of Justice. Los Angeles Pharmacist Sentenced to 18 months in Prison for Medicare Part D Scheme. Washington, DC: US Department of Justice; 2015. Accessed May 21, 2021. https://www.justice.gov/opa/pr/los-angeles-pharmacist-sentenced-18-months-prison-medicare-part-d-scheme

31. Centers for Medicare and Medicaid Services (CMS). Medicaid Fraud & Abuse: Prevent, Detect, Report. Baltimore, MD: CMS; 2019. Accessed May 21, 2021. https://www.cms.gov/Outreach-and-Education/Medicare-Learning-Network-MLN/MLNProducts/Downloads/Fraud-Abuse-MLN4649244.pdf

32. Department of Justice. Iserve Technologies, Inc. Pled Guilty in Connection with Guilty Pleas of Former Exec and Manager of Med-Fast Pharmacy Inc. Washington, DC: US Department of Justice; 2017. Accessed May 21, 2021. https://www.justice.gov/usao-wdpa/pr/iserve-technologies-inc-pled-guilty-connection-guilty-pleas-former-exec-and-manager-med

33. 42 USC §1320a-7b(a).

34. 42 CFR §1001.952.

35. US Department of Justice. Justice News. Accessed May 21, 2021. https://www.justice.gov/news

36. 42 USC §1395nn.

37. 42 CFR §411.357.

38. 42 USC §1395nn(g).

39. Department of Justice. Justice Department Recovers over $3 Billion for False Claims Act Cases in Fiscal Year 2019. Washington, DC: 2020. Accessed May 21, 2021. https://www.justice.gov/opa/pr/justice-department-recovers-over-3-billion-false-claims-act-cases-fiscal-year-2019

40. 21 CFR §1306.11.

41. 45 CFR §164.524.

42. 45 CFR §164.512.

# 6

# PHARMACY INVENTORY

*Jeremy Ashley, PharmD, and Mark Sullivan, BPharm*

---

## ▨ LEARNING OBJECTIVES

1. Compare and contrast wholesale versus direct drug purchasing processes and strategies.
2. Describe the implementation and requirements for the Drug Supply Chain Security Act (DSCSA).
3. Explain pharmacy storage requirements and organization recommendations.
4. List inventory management and legal recordkeeping requirements.

You have been a practicing pharmacist for the last 5 years. Your current role is a staff pharmacist at a regional grocery store chain pharmacy. The pharmacy you serve is one of the top performing stores in the company with weekly sales averaging over $250 000 and a prescription volume of 5000 scripts per week. The pharmacy's existing inventory totals over $1 million. The current Pharmacist-in-Charge or Pharmacy Manager is relocating across the state and you have been offered the position. You don't have any pharmacy management experience, but your past performance and hard work makes your Regional Director of Pharmacy confident that you are the right person for the job. After accepting the job, you take over as Pharmacist-in-Charge in 1 week. You have also been informed by your Regional Director that your pharmacy is due to take inventory in 1 month. Feeling clueless about pharmacy inventory and its management, you spend some time talking with the current Pharmacist-in-Charge.

## ■ WHAT IS PHARMACY INVENTORY?

In a strict definition, pharmacy inventory is the product that is available and in saleable or usable condition within your pharmacy. Pharmacy inventory may include nonsalable items such as out-of-date products or recalled items not yet processed. This includes pharmaceutical ingredients used in compounding.

Beyond this strict definition, pharmacy inventory can be expanded to include the purchasing options, requirements, regulations, and recordkeeping associated with the products mentioned above. In this chapter, we will explore all the components of pharmacy inventory.

## ■ DRUG PURCHASING

Drug purchasing is one of the most important, yet a complex issue in managing a pharmacy. Inventory is generally a pharmacy's largest asset and drug purchasing is the key to driving cash flow and profitability to the bottom line. With the wide variety of purchasing options, terms, and ordering methods available today, finding the right mix for the individual pharmacy is imperative to proper inventory control and profitability.

If you were opening or managing a pharmacy today, there would be several choices you would have to make regarding how to procure your inventory. These decisions must be made to provide the most efficient and profitable method of sourcing your inventory.

### Purchasing Options

First, where do you buy your inventory?

You have several options available to you, but the most common is to buy through a *purchase agreement* with a *drug wholesaler* such as AmerisourceBergen®, Cardinal®, or McKesson® to name a few. A primary wholesale account can be set up with a wholesaler to allow you to order products on a daily basis at a contracted purchase price. To provide redundancy for shortages or other more specific reasons, a secondary account can be set up with a different wholesaler that fits your needs. You may have more than 2 wholesalers but the more access points you add in your supply chain, the more difficult it becomes to manage. There are numerous secondary wholesalers that specialize in different segments of pharmacy business such as generics, specialty items, or short-dated products.

Another option would be to buy *direct* from the manufacturer. This avenue generally takes a large volume of drug movement to make it financially feasible for the manufacturer as well as for the pharmacy. This can become very cumbersome when managing accounts across multiple manufacturers that may have different policies, minimum orders, and contract terms. *Direct purchasing* is normally reserved for larger pharmacy groups and those maintaining their own warehouses. Some pharmacies, however, may use this method when procuring specific product categories such as vaccines.

## Wholesaler Terms

When setting up a primary wholesale purchasing account, a contract must be signed that will delineate all the responsibilities of both parties under that specific purchasing agreement. Inside of the agreement, the terms of purchase will be defined. These terms include the brand name contract pricing, generic contract pricing, returns policies, payment terms, and other pertinent items. Pricing terms can be defined in several ways but are generally represented as a discount off of the *average wholesale price* or the *wholesale acquisition cost*. This will depend on the wholesaler and the negotiated discount offer. Many wholesalers will offer monthly, quarterly, and yearly rebate reductions of invoice pricing as a concession for volume, brand/generic purchasing ratios, generic preferred contract compliance, and overall spend.

Many other items in addition to pricing should be negotiated in these contracts. These will include items such as return policies, payment terms, delivery schedules, special pricing for unique categories, seasonal offers, and other non-drug products and services that wholesalers may offer.

## Group Purchasing Organization (GPO) Affiliations

Another option for pharmacies is to join a *group purchasing organization (GPO)*. By joining a GPO, you combine your volume and purchasing power with other similar pharmacies to provide greater leverage in contract negotiations. The downside is that you would have to give up control of the negotiations to the controlling body of the GPO. The GPO will negotiate all terms we have discussed and also will handle the bidding for the supplier or wholesaler that will be chosen to service the group for the term of the contract. In many cases this is a very good option, especially for small groups, independents, and hospitals.

## Ordering Methods

Finally, you need to decide on the method you will use to order each day.

The first method to order is referred to as *order-by-use*. This process is accomplished by adding to the daily open order each time you empty a stock bottle or use a *unit-of-use* product during the dispensing process. This is a manual process and leaves the possibility for human error.

The second method, known as *replenishment*, is similar to the *by-use* method. This is a process where your dispensing system creates a daily order based on the full package sizes of all products dispensed during the day. This order can be generated and submitted electronically but still gives you less fine control over your inventory management.

The third method is to reorder by established *reorder points (ROP)* or *periodic automatic replenishment (PAR)* level. This requires a little more upfront setup by the pharmacy staff in setting up and maintaining a perpetual inventory, to ensure accuracy of orders. These orders are automatically generated when the inventory level falls below the ROP or PAR value set up for that drug.

The last order method is known as *just-in-time* ordering. This is a process when you order a product only when it is needed. Some use this method to keep their inventory levels low and have less inventory on the shelves at risk (high cost, short expiration dates, low prescription volume, etc.). This method has a larger chance of out of stocks and lost sales from product availability. This method is also dependent on the reliability of your supplier and your delivery.

## ■ DRUG SUPPLY CHAIN SECURITY ACT: "TRACK AND TRACE"

The Drug Quality and Security Act (DQSA) was enacted by Congress on November 27, 2013. Title II of DQSA, the Drug Supply Chain Security Act (DSCSA), outlines the steps for creation of an electronic system to identify and trace prescription drugs as they are distributed in the United States supply chain.[1–3] This system will enhance the ability to help protect consumers from exposure to drugs that may be counterfeit, stolen, contaminated, or dangerous to the public. The system will also improve detection and removal of potentially dangerous drugs from the drug supply chain to protect consumers.

In addition, the DSCSA directs the FDA to establish national standards for manufacturers, re-packagers, wholesale distributors, third-party logistics providers, and pharmacies to ensure the goals of the act are met.

DSCSA is not intended to be a full "track and trace" program as some may think. This program was designed to standardize the documentation of each supply chain event, so items could be easily identified and investigated if there ever were a problem that required intervention. Most products or transactions in the supply chain will never be verified because of this. The documentation for each step in the supply chain requires each participant to provide three pieces of transactional data: transactional information (TI), transaction history (TH), and a transactional statement (TS) from the previous owner to be supplied to each subsequent owner. Each owner must maintain their transactional data for every transaction for a period of 6 years.

The timeline for implementation of DSCSA began with enactment in 2013 and will complete with the last required step in November of 2023.[4] Here is a brief overview of each step.

*January 1, 2015*
DSCSA began by requiring all pharmaceutical manufacturers to print lot numbers on packaging for all prescription drugs.

*November 27, 2018*
DSCSA required pharmaceutical manufacturers and re-packagers to include unique serial numbers and expiration dates on prescription drug packaging. This information had to be in a human-readable format and in GS1 barcodes as well as inclusion in 2D codes (Data Matrix Codes). Manufacturers and re-packagers also had to capture and store TI, TH, and TS in their databases for at least 6 years.

*November 27, 2019*
Pharmaceutical wholesalers must authenticate and verify prescription drugs before reselling them. They must only buy and sell products with serial numbers and the right barcodes, as well as capture TI, TH, and TS for creating proper documents for product tracking. They are also required to authenticate and verify saleable returns using the Verification Router Service.

*November 27, 2020*
Dispensers will need to authenticate and verify all the medications they buy before selling them to consumers. They will need to store all TI, TH, and TS data for product tracking and tracing.

*November 27, 2023*
By the end of 2023, the entire supply chain must be DSCSA compliant. Complete unit-level traceability, including aggregation, will be mandatory. Aggregation is the process by which data relationships are established between unique identifiers of saleable units, the cartons into which they are packed, and the next level of packaging, cases, and pallets allowing full traceability down to the unit level.

The requirements for community pharmacy began in November 2020.[4] To become fully compliant, pharmacies will need to capture and maintain all transactional data on each product that they buy or sell. When a pharmacy sells a prescription, they must attach their dispensing data to the lot number and expiration date of each prescription that is sold. This data must be maintained for a period of 6 years. To achieve this, pharmacies must only buy from sources that can provide this required transactional data with each purchase. In addition, pharmacy software must also apply the actual lot and expiration dates of each unit dispensed in each prescription. For example, when a prescription is dispensed from 2 different stock bottles, both sets of serialization will need to be recorded with the details of that prescription.

In conclusion, DSCSA means serialization, aggregation, and exchanging transaction information, in addition to authentication for recalls, resales, and returns, along with risk-based intervention for each suspected product, to ensure that only safe medications are dispensed to the public.

# PHARMACY ENVIRONMENT AND INVENTORY STORAGE AND ORGANIZATION

A *Pharmacist-in-Charge (PIC)* is challenged with carrying the responsibility of operating a successful business, as well as ensuring that the behind-the-scenes duties and tasks of the pharmacy are taken care of. There is an old saying that "you are only as strong as your weakest link," and the same is true in pharmacy business today. Maintaining the pharmacy environment and inventory requires a complete team effort. Creating pharmacy checklists and assigning daily duties to pharmacy employees are some examples of ways to preserve the pharmacy workplace. The purpose of this section is to provide general guidance for these concepts to efficiently maintain and dispense reliable medications from your pharmacy.

## Pharmacy Environment

The PIC is responsible for ensuring that the pharmacy is clean and orderly with all equipment in good working condition. It is critical for the pharmacy to have proper lighting and be well ventilated. The temperature of the pharmacy and the pharmacy refrigerator/freezer needs to be maintained within a range compatible with the proper storage of drugs.

Many state agencies and pharmacy organizations define temperature by the following *United States Pharmacopeia (USP)* definitions:[5]

1. Room temperature: the ambient temperature in a work area
2. Controlled room temperature storage requirement: 20–25 °C (68–77 °F)
3. Cool storage requirement: 8–15 °C (46–59 °F)
4. Refrigerator storage requirement: 2–8 °C (36–46 °F)
5. Freezer storage requirement: −25 °C to −10 °C (−13 °F to 14 °F)

Humidity-monitoring devices should be used in cases where repackaged medications are humidity-sensitive or labeled to avoid moisture. USP defines a dry place as one that does not exceed 40% average relative humidity at controlled room temperature of the equivalent water vapor pressure at other temperatures.

The PIC is responsible for maintaining pharmacy security requirements and confirming effective protocols are in place to guard against theft and diversion of controlled substances. Some security controls include the following:

1. Pharmacy alarm systems are activated and tested regularly.
2. Locked closures on vaults, safes, and secure cabinets are consistently validated.
3. Pharmacy access is monitored and key control systems are maintained.

## Inventory Storage and Organization

The majority of the time, the pharmacy inventory is the most expensive component of a pharmacy's business. For some pharmacies, a drug inventory could easily total over a million dollars. When thinking about a large chain pharmacy, that total dollar amount could potentially reach the billions when adding all of the individual store's inventories together. The PIC having knowledge of the pharmacy's inventory and maintaining its storage and organization is key to a successful business.

To begin, all prescription drugs and devices should be stored within the pharmacy or in a locked storage area at the proper temperature as defined by the USP.[5]

Drug inventories are commonly organized within the pharmacy shelves alphabetically by a drug's brand or generic name. Some commonly dispensed drugs may have a special shelf close to the dispensing area called a "fast movers" section. These drugs have high dispensing rates and being close to the dispensing area improves workflow efficiency.

Depending on the state of practice, controlled substances may require extra attention. Federal law states that pharmacies may store controlled substances listed in Schedule II through Schedule V in a securely locked, substantially constructed cabinet or they may be dispersed throughout noncontrolled substance stock in a manner that will obstruct theft.[6] When comparing state and federal law regarding controlled substances, it is important to ensure the stricter law is enforced.

Conducting inventory *cycle counts* often helps maintain the pharmacy inventory. Cycle counts are defined as a procedure where a small subset or category of drugs is counted at a specific time. The PIC should conduct cycle counts of Schedule II through Schedule V and other high-risk or high-dollar drugs deemed necessary on a scheduled basis. The interval for this type of cycle count could be mandated by state law or a company policy. Cycle counts are different from traditional inventory in·that it is less disruptive to daily operations, provides an ongoing measure of inventory accuracy and procedure execution, and can be medication-specific.

Drug inventory should be checked regularly to ensure no expired drugs or devices are on the pharmacy shelves. Out-of-date drugs cannot be dispensed beyond the expiration date and must be removed from dispensing stock. Out-of-date drugs must be separated from active stock until disposal and removal from the pharmacy. Best practice is to rotate drug stock by making sure products with approaching expiration dates are front-facing and dispensed before products with later expiration dates. For business purposes, remember that if a drug has expired, it cannot be sold; therefore, profit from a sale cannot be generated.

## ■ INVENTORY MANAGEMENT: LEGAL AND RECORDKEEPING

The task of taking any inventory in a community pharmacy can be stressful and overwhelming for the PIC. As you can imagine, the drugs that get the most attention during inventory are controlled substances (Schedules II, III, IV, and V). The key to having a successful inventory conducted in short amount of time requires the following:

1. Identifying efficient technicians and preparing a team to help conduct the inventory.
2. Become familiar with your state's specific inventory requirements (as they may be stricter than the federal requirements).
3. Taking some time before the scheduled inventory to prepare. Inventory preparation may include organizing prescription shelves, cleaning, and separating expired medications (while separating controlled substances from legend drugs).

### General Inventory Requirements

The PIC's presence is required for taking pharmacy inventory, although tasks may be delegated to another pharmacy employee. The inventory record is maintained in written, typewritten, or printed form.[7] If inventory is verbally recorded, the outcome must be promptly transcribed.[7]

The inventory record is kept in the pharmacy and available for inspection for at least 2 years and is filed separately from all other pharmacy records.[7] The inventory record needs to include all stocks of controlled substances on hand on the date of inventory (including any which are out of date).[7]

The inventory can be taken before the pharmacy opens for business or after the pharmacy closes for business on the inventory date.[7] The inventory record indicates whether the inventory is taken as of the opening of business or as of the close of business on the inventory date (if the pharmacy is open 24 hours a day, then the time that the inventory was taken is documented).[7]

The person(s) taking the inventory conducts an exact count of all controlled substances listed in Schedule II.[7] The person(s) taking the inventory conducts an estimated count or measure of all controlled substances listed in Schedules III, IV, and V unless the container holds more than 1000 tablets or capsules, in which case, an exact count of the contents must be made.[7]

The inventory of Schedule II controlled substances is listed separately from the inventory of

Schedules III, IV, and V controlled substances.[7] If the pharmacy maintains a perpetual inventory of any of the drugs required to be inventoried, the perpetual inventory shall be reconciled on the date of inventory.[7]

### Reasons for Taking Inventory

There are six reasons why a pharmacy would take an inventory:

1. Required before a new pharmacy opens for business (considered an initial inventory).[7]
2. Federal law requires an inventory to be completed every 2 years (a biennial inventory) after the date on which the initial inventory was taken.[7]
   a. The PIC must reconcile the 2-year federal requirement with the state requirement, as many states have additional or stricter requirements regarding inventories for controlled substances.
   b. Remember, always follow the stricter law. Let's look at Texas law for an example. Texas requires an annual inventory of all controlled substances on hand on May 1 of each year or on the pharmacy's regular general physical inventory date.[8] Such inventory may be taken within 4 days of the specified inventory. This annual inventory must contain records of the employee and PIC participating via signature, the time the inventory was taken, and date the inventory with the date it was taken. The signature of the PIC and the date of inventory must be notarized within 3 business days of the day the inventory is completed.[8]
   c. Some chain pharmacy companies may have stricter inventory policies. One company may require a biennial inventory, where another company may require a quarterly inventory.
3. Change of ownership of a pharmacy (includes Class A Community Pharmacy).[7]
4. Closing of a pharmacy.[7]
5. Change of PIC.[7]
6. When a drug is newly scheduled by the DEA.[7]

## ■ CHAPTER APPLICATIONS

1. At the beginning of this chapter (Setting the Scene), you learned that a promotion is in your near future. As the incoming PIC, what questions would you have for the current PIC regarding pharmacy inventory and its management?
2. Understanding how to purchase inventory in the most efficient and effective manner is one of the leading drivers to the profitability of a pharmacy. Using what we have discussed above, you should now be able to make the appropriate choices for any situation you find yourself in. Consider the pharmacies where you have been on rotation or worked throughout your training and list the inventory purchasing options and methods for each location. Which did you think were the most effective?
3. Pharmacists, or "dispensers" under the DSCSA, need to know their responsibilities under the DSCSA to protect patients from receiving harmful drug products. The DSCSA includes requirements that pharmacies must follow to protect patients from receiving harmful drugs, such as counterfeit or other illegitimate drugs. What actions are required by pharmacies under the DSCSA when a prescription is sold?
4. Your pharmacy's production is exceeding your current workspace and is eligible for remodel which will double the size of your current space. After construction is finished and you are able to move into the new pharmacy space, what are some things to consider when relocating and organizing your current pharmacy inventory?
5. It is time for your pharmacy to take inventory. Make a checklist of inventory requirements and to-do items that will help you conduct a successful inventory.

# REFERENCES

1. Drug Supply Chain Security Act. Section. 202. Pharmaceutical Distribution Supply Chain. Chapter V (21 USC §351 et seq.).
2. Department of Health and Human Services. The Drug Supply Chain Security Act Implementation: Product Tracing Requirements for Dispensers—Compliance Policy. Federal Register. 2015;80(128):38449–38450. Published July 6, 2015. Accessed September 8, 2020. gpo.gov/fdsys/pkg/FR-2015-07-06/pdf/2015-16401.pdf
3. Department of Health and Human Services. The Drug Supply Chain Security Act Implementation: Product Tracing Requirements for Dispensers-Compliance Policy; Updated Guidance for Industry, Availability. Published November 2, 2015. Accessed May 25, 2021. https://www.federalregister.gov/documents/2015/11/02/2015-27841/the-drug-supply-chain-security-act-implementation-product-tracing-requirements-for
4. The Pew Charitable Trusts. Pharmacy Implementation of the Drug Supply Chain Security Act. Published September, 2014. Accessed May 25, 2021. pewtrusts.org/~/media/assets/2014/09/dsp_drugsafety_dcscafactsheet_v2.pdf
5. US Pharmacopeial Convention. Accessed May 25, 2021. https://www.usp.org
6. 21 CFR §1301.75.
7. 21 CFR §1304.11.
8. TAC §291.17.

# 7

# ROLE OF TECHNOLOGY IN COMMUNITY PHARMACY

*Lance Thompson, PharmD, Vanessa Brown, PharmD, and Will Douglas, PharmD*

---

### ■ LEARNING OBJECTIVES

1. Describe the types of technology utilized in the community pharmacy setting.
2. Discuss how technology can be used to optimize community pharmacy operations and patient care.
3. Explain the use of technology solutions to address problems in the community pharmacy setting.

## ■ SETTING THE SCENE

The profession of pharmacy has come a long way since the days of herbalist healers in ancient Babylon. Remedies for all sorts of maladies that were once inscribed onto clay tablets are now prescribed entirely digital. Many processes that were paper-based even a decade ago are now done online. In the past, concerns about HIPAA and other regulations, while legitimate, slowed the development of new technology in pharmacy. However, current market forces, including the COVID-19 pandemic, and patient demand have led to a flourishing environment for new technology solutions within community pharmacy.

We will discuss specific tools and programs and highlight their uses to address problems or inefficiencies seen in the community pharmacy setting. As you read about the different tools, remember that technology should never replace your clinical expertise. Technology exists to assist you, not replace you. Many of the tools discussed in this chapter provide increased time for pharmacists to focus on soft skills. It is your responsibility to harness these tools to improve patient care and improve your pharmacy operations.

## ■ HOW DOES TECHNOLOGY HELP PATIENTS?

Patient demand for convenience has driven many of the advances in technology for pharmacy. For example, within the last few years, pharmacy software programs have developed capabilities for pharmacists to converse with patients via text directly from the software. Fifteen years ago, most in our profession would have thought this impossible due to Health Insurance Portability and Accountability Act of 1996 (HIPAA) regulations and technology limitations, but the best solutions found a way. This is a common theme with any technological development; if the market demands it, the solution will eventually develop.

Let's discuss some of the prominent technological developments that help patients:

- Online and Mobile Application-based Refills
  - These methods solve problems for both patients and providers by streamlining refill requests. This reduces phone calls which is a huge benefit to pharmacy staff.
- Communication Tools
  - Text messaging and reminders
    - Many patients can now text their pharmacists directly. This, combined with automated refill and pickup reminders, provides a convenient way for patients to stay connected and compliant.
  - Telepharmacy and video-based counseling
    - In 2020, many pharmacies quickly adapted to using new tools to fulfill their clinical responsibilities while adhering to SARS-CoV-2 and Coronavirus 2019 (COVID-19) precautions and regulations. One such way was utilizing video-based counseling tools for patients who had their medications delivered to their homes. There are several different options for this, including telepharmacy built into pharmacy software programs. The benefit is they replicate the traditional face-to-face counseling interaction but allow patients to do so from wherever they choose.
- Scheduling Platforms
  - During the COVID-19 pandemic, software companies began offering HIPAA-compliant websites for patients to schedule immunization appointments. Some sites even integrated directly with pharmacy software platforms to improve pharmacy workflow.
  - Many patients and pharmacies benefited from these tools as they simplified the patient intake process while also providing convenient appointment reminders.
  - Patient scheduling websites will likely continue to thrive even after COVID-19, as options to schedule flu shots or MedSync appointments will still be desirable.

- Delivery Advancements
  - Delivery has been a common practice, especially among independent community pharmacies. However, medication delivery has expanded with third-party companies like Zipdrug® and Uber® specifically completing that task for patients.
- Medication Synchronization (med sync)
  - Whether you are using a third-party vendor or your current pharmacy management software, this program helps to synchronize medications for patients. Medication synchronization is when the pharmacist coordinates medication refills so the patient can pick them up on a single day each month. This eliminates the need to call in multiple prescription refills and may help increase patient's medication adherence and the pharmacy's bottom line.
- Wearable Technology
  - Heart rate monitors, continuous glucose monitors, and other wearable monitors are becoming easier to use and can transmit data directly to the patient's healthcare providers. Some smartwatches can even perform multiple monitoring functions as opposed to using a separate device for each function. The data from a patient's wearable device can be immensely useful to pharmacists for disease state management.
- Pharmacogenomics (PGx)
  - As PGx becomes more commonplace, more patients will gain insight into how their genetic makeup affects the way they may respond to the medications they take. In the last two decades, this technology has become more readily available to patients. Reporting has become easier and costs have steadily declined. PGx can save patients time, money, and potentially adverse health effects. Pharmacists are well suited to help patients navigate the complex information provided by PGx results.
- Amazon®, PillPack®, Roman®, and others
  - With the advent of direct-to-consumer pharmacies like Roman®, TruePill®, and Pillpack®, the pharmacy landscape is changing. Segmentation is now common, which increases the risk of polypharmacy. Amazon's purchase of Pillpack®, which was a startup only a few years earlier, further shows that our profession is ripe for disruption. Many community pharmacies must now compete with these online businesses daily for patients.
- Blockchain and Data Unions
  - Blockchains are defined by Merriam-Webster as a "digital database containing information … that can be simultaneously used and shared within a large decentralized, publicly accessible network blockchain."[1] The term is a buzzword for multiple industries, but it is a productive tool when wielded correctly. The two following examples help paint a picture of the different ways patients can benefit from this technology.
    - New programs like RemediChain match patients who need specific, high-cost medications with other patients who no longer need them through a donation program. This is established securely through a ledger-based system that connects the two parties, with a pharmacy in the middle as a secure distributor.
    - Data unions may rise in the future so patients could participate in long-term studies based on their health and medication regimens, especially if the data is combined with wearables. This could allow patients to control how their health data is used and potentially be compensated for it.[2]

## ■ HOW DOES TECHNOLOGY HELP A PHARMACY AND BUSINESS?

There is a litany of tasks that must be performed in the pharmacy each day. Some are simple, others are complex. Yet, nearly all of them must be done while complying with HIPAA and ensuring data integrity.

Technology solutions can expedite many of these tasks and free up staff for other important responsibilities. Let's look at some of the options available to community pharmacies:

- Automatic Counting Devices (ACDs)
  - ACDs free up pharmacists and staff from the burden of hand-counting prescriptions. Some devices can automate up to 95% of countable prescriptions while other counting devices help to identify potential errors during a manual counting process.[3]
  - Some examples of ACDs are Eyecon, Kirby Lester, and Parata.
    - Eyecon devices visually count tablets using a camera and can record pictures of the counted medication for documentation.
    - Kirby Lester devices are commonly used when counting larger quantities of drugs to expedite the process.
    - Parata and other "robots," as they are called in many pharmacies, are typically filled with the common drugs or "fast-movers." When prescriptions are entered for these drugs, the robotic counting machine automatically fills the proper quantity, and many machines can label and cap the vial also. Some automated counting machines can count and process blister-packed medications as well.
- Central Fill Service
  - Central fill is a program where one main filling pharmacy enters into an agreement with one or more pharmacies, and that main filling pharmacy counts, vials, and labels the prescriptions for the others.[4] This efficiently reduces the majority of the burden of filling scripts for the other pharmacies.
- Compliance and Data Integrity
  - Protecting patient privacy and data security is paramount in today's information age. Many technology programs contain multiple safeguards to comply with local company policies as well as state and federal regulations.
- Controlled Substance Ordering System (CSOS) and CSOS cloud
  - This technology allows a pharmacy to digitally meet all the Drug Enforcement Administration (DEA) requirements for ordering schedule two medications without the supporting paper DEA Form 222. Using a technology called public key infrastructure, CSOS requires that each individual purchaser enrolls with the DEA to acquire a CSOS digital certificate.[5]
  - Some wholesalers took this a step further and used cloud-based technology to create CSOS Cloud. This program allows a pharmacy to order schedule II from any registered device.
- Pharmacy Software Programs
  - Many of the other things you've read about in this chapter, as well as in this book (inventory management, clinical tools) are encompassed within pharmacy software programs.
  - While chain drug stores have proprietary programs, independent pharmacies may choose from several options. Many of the programs have built-in tools like electronic purchase orders, eCare plans, and clinical alerts.
  - Some pharmacy software programs also integrate with third-party companies to provide a full suite of tools to users. The future of these programs is rapidly evolving in this competitive market, and pharmacists stand to benefit greatly from new developments.
- Prescription Drug Monitoring Programs (PDMPs)
  - An electronic database that is managed by states and tracks controlled substance dispensing. These platforms provide timely information to help pharmacists and other healthcare professionals perform their professional responsibility of improving opioid prescribing and identifying patients at risk.[6]
  - Before PDMPs were established, a pharmacist had to rely on their instinct, patient red flags, and insurance rejections for duplicate therapy to help them determine whether a patient was at risk of addiction or seeing multiple doctors and multiple pharmacies. Those with their "detective hats" on would spend precious time chasing down suspicious leads only to get further behind in their workload as they wait on hold. Now it is a simple verification process to help you stay compliant and keep your patients safe.
- Remote Prescription Processing
  - This technology allows prescriptions to be processed by pharmacists who are not present on-site. This can improve workflow by allowing pools of

pharmacists to verify scripts on-demand. It can also help pharmacies in more rural communities access pharmacist verification services more easily.

## HOW DOES TECHNOLOGY HELP PHARMACISTS?

Each day in the pharmacy, you are likely to interact with numerous types of technology. Using these tools effectively can help you to practice at the top of your license. Let's take a look:

- Clinical Alerts
  - Each day you work in the pharmacy you will likely receive numerous notifications for drug-drug or drug-disease interactions. When a patient has a drug or disease interaction, an alert will pop up in your prescription processing software to warn you. Additionally, you may also get notified if the patient is eligible for age-specific vaccinations, like the shingles vaccine.
  - It is important to not be worn down by these (aka alert fatigue) and to take them seriously. It is also important to remember that your clinical judgment takes precedence. You should know your patients and their medical history enough to make more informed decisions than your computer.
- eCare Plans
  - These are a relatively new development for community pharmacists to engage and document clinical interventions with patients. Many independent pharmacies participate in these, intending to aggregate enough data to show meaningful pharmacist interventions.
  - Some pharmacy software programs include eCare documentation directly within the program. Other companies offer eCare plans within their suite of other services that integrate with the pharmacy software programs.
- Medication Therapy Management (MTM)
  - Many software platforms integrate with MTM programs like OutcomesMTM®. This allows

pharmacists to easily manage immunizations, chronic diseases, and other MTM priorities directly from their software or online website. That means more MTM opportunities can be completed without the added burden of documenting on multiple software platforms.
- Point-of-Care Testing Solutions
  - Just like immunizations, pharmacies have an opportunity to own part of this market. With more advances in this area, equipment is becoming more affordable with better functionality and accuracy of results. Pharmacies can provide services on-site for acute and chronic care testing such as Group A streptococcal pharyngitis, influenza, COVID-19, INR, hepatitis C, cholesterol, and HbA1c, right inside the pharmacy.

## CONCLUSION

It is important to remember that technology should augment, but not replace your judgment as a community pharmacist. It is also important to evaluate the newest technology from multiple perspectives. The simplest way to understand how technology may change is to look at any process you currently do and ask "what would this look like if it were easy?" Who knows, if you think about it hard enough, you may provide the next big solution in pharmacy technology.

## CHAPTER APPLICATIONS

1. A patient is inconsistent with measuring their blood pressure daily, despite being advised by their physician to do so. They lament this fact to you while picking up their refills for their current medications. What technology solutions can you suggest to help them monitor their blood pressure more easily?
2. You notice Shirley has come into the pharmacy for the third time already this month. As you are ringing her up you mention you've noticed

her frequent visits. She complains that she can't keep up with when it is time to refill her medications. She is frustrated with how often she has to visit the pharmacy and wishes she could get all her prescriptions at one time. What technology solutions can you offer to help the patient?

3. You have a patient that is inconsistent with refilling and picking up their medications on time. What technology solutions are available to help this situation?

4. You have a loyal patient coming in with a prescription for a hydrocodone/acetaminophen 5/325 mg, a Schedule II pain medication, for his mother that is in hospice. You do not have the product in stock and need to order it quickly, but your pharmacy manager is off duty this weekend and lives far away from the pharmacy. What technology solutions could you use for this patient without sending them to another pharmacy?

5. You receive a prescription for a patient for meloxicam 15 mg, once daily. When verifying the prescription, a clinical warning pops up on your screen as a major interaction between the meloxicam, and the new prescription from the patient's dentist for ibuprofen 800 mg TID × 7 days from 6 months ago. What should you do to address this drug interaction alert?

## REFERENCES

1. Merriam-Webster. Blockchain. Accessed April 7, 2021. https://www.merriam-webster.com/dictionary/blockchain
2. Miller R. Data Unions. Robert Miller's Blog. Published August 24, 2018. Accessed April 7, 2021. bertcmiller.com/2018/08/24/data-unions.html
3. High Drug Volume Dispensing System. McKesson. Accessed September 20, 2020. https://www.mckesson.com/Pharmacy-Management/Automation/Automated-Drug-Dispensing/
4. Centralized Pharmacy Prescription Dispensing Service. McKesson. Accessed September 20, 2020. www.mckesson.com/Pharmacy-Management/Automation/Central-Fill-Service/
5. CSOS Overview. E-Commerce Program. Drug Enforcement Administration. Diversion Control Division. Accessed September 19, 2020. https://www.deaecom.gov/about.html
6. Prescription Drug Monitoring Programs. Centers for Disease Control and Prevention. Accessed September 20, 2020. https://www.cdc.gov/drugoverdose/pdmp/states.html

# 8

# PROFIT, LOSS, AND RISK MANAGEMENT

*Kenneth C. Hohmeier, PharmD, and Donald C. Hohmeier, CPA-Retired*

---

## ▓ LEARNING OBJECTIVES

1. Define key terms used for financial analysis and accounting.
2. Describe the two major financial statements used to assess a pharmacy's financial and operational performance.
3. Describe where "the bottom line" of a pharmacy's financial performance is found.
4. Describe what is meant by "risk" and how a pharmacy may mitigate it.
5. Provide tools to better manage a pharmacy and clearly communicate with pharmacy personnel, advisors, and other stakeholders.

## ■ SETTING THE SCENE

You have just been promoted to co-manager of a new pharmacy in a large national pharmacy chain. One of your new responsibilities is to review business reports generated by your regional manager and by the pharmacy software system on a periodic basis. Your regional manager expects you to create action plans based on these reports. The pharmacy manager expects frequent updates and has also requested that you provide a high-level overview of how the pharmacy is performing financially and operationally. The company's accounting firm visits on occasion and seems to be speaking a different language. You feel a bit overwhelmed. Although some of the reports make sense to you to read, you do not feel comfortable enough with any of the reports to explain the results to others.

## ■ WHAT IS PROFIT, LOSS, AND RISK MANAGEMENT?

Whether you are a pharmacist in a chain or independent community pharmacy, understanding your business's finances is critically important for pharmacy success—and ultimately patient care. It must also be noted that familiarity with financial reporting and analysis should not be solely reserved for the pharmacy manager, leader, or owner. At a minimum, every pharmacist should have a baseline understanding of financial basics, including profit, loss, and risk management. For a front-line pharmacist, it may allow you to advocate for a new patient care service in terms of dollars and cents—a language more likely to be understood in making the case for that service. As a pharmacy manager, this will give you the tools to review and assess the various reports available to you so that you can understand, plan, and improve the pharmacy's business. This is similar to collecting and analyzing patient care data, such as laboratory results, and then forming a patient care plan. Just as one must communicate in the same language as their patients to ensure understanding if they are going to provide

optimal patient care, a community pharmacist too, must understand the language of finance if they are going to optimize the impact of their pharmacy on their community.

A pharmacist is first and foremost a clinician. Although in the United States, the doctor of pharmacy degree confers some basic understanding of business management and leadership as required by the Accreditation Council for Pharmacy Education (ACPE), it does not make such knowledge the priority.[1] In this same spirit, this chapter presents information with an understanding that the goal is not to make the reader an expert in finance, but rather a pharmacy expert who is able to communicate easily and correctly with those who *are* financial experts. Moreover, it is the goal of this chapter to provide community pharmacists baseline skills to read and assess financial reports common to a community pharmacy. Finally, readers can use the information in this chapter to improve the way they communicate community pharmacy goals, strategies, and other business-related metrics and their importance to front line pharmacy support staff (i.e., pharmacy technicians, cashiers, and part-time pharmacists.) These stakeholders may be less interested in finance, but are likely very interested in the financial health and well-being of the organization for which they work. Translating key financial ideas, reports, and updates into easily understandable highlights will help the entire community pharmacy team function in a more cohesive unit.

## ■ ACCOUNTING

Core to understanding finance is understanding the profession responsible for its standards, best practices, and general practice. Like "pharmacy," "accounting" refers to both a profession and a practice. As a community pharmacist you can and will perform some basic accounting at your pharmacy; however, ultimately an accountant is going to be the expert who you and your organization will rely on for the health of the business and regulatory compliance.

Accountants bring much value to the business of pharmacy. It is most often your accountant who will assemble your pharmacy's raw financial records into standard financial reports. Your accountant may be a Certified Public Accountant (CPA), a credential indicating that he or she has met the state's rigorous education and experience requirements. However, all accountants must follow a standard set of rules known as Generally Accepted Accounting Principles (GAAP), which assures uniformity of recording transactions and reporting activity across all industries, as well as brings consistency and credibility to those stakeholders who rely on the accuracy of the reports (i.e., owners, investors, and financial institutions). Accountants are proficient in analyzing your financial reports and can help you understand how your pharmacy is performing relative to its past results or the industry overall. Perhaps most importantly, your accountant can offer suggestions for improving your business operations and help you prepare plans and budgets to act as a roadmap for your pharmacy's future financial success.

Lastly, your accountant will likely plan for, prepare, and file the pharmacy's income, payroll, and other business tax returns. The complexity of the various federal, state, and local tax codes places this topic well beyond the scope of this chapter. Your accountant's understanding of your business and the applicable tax laws make him or her particularly qualified to act as your "trusted adviser," and you should consult with them for any tax advice.

## ■ FINANCE BASICS AND TERMINOLOGY

For those just beginning to learn and apply finance principles, it is essential to "speak the correct language." Often in our personal lives we use terms like "income," "profit," "debt," and others—but these colloquial definitions usually differ in subtle and not-so-subtle ways from definitions used in the finance world. There is no easier way to confuse your coworkers and colleagues in accounting and financial management than to use the wrong word; for instance, to say

"profit" when you mean "revenue." Most importantly, understanding these terms will allow pharmacists to understand and assess the *financial statements*, covered after this section.[2,3]

In this section we will define the terms *asset, liability, equity, revenue* (or *income* or *sales*), *cost of goods sold (COGS), gross profit, expense*, and *profit* (or *net income*).

*Assets* are simply items owned by a pharmacy. Some examples of these include property such as computers, prescription, and over-the-counter (OTC) inventory, benches, chairs, and shelving. Cash and customer accounts receivable (money owed to the pharmacy) are also assets. If the pharmacy owns its own building, this would be an asset as well.

*Liabilities* are somewhat the reverse of an asset. Whereas an asset represents value for the organization, a liability represents something owed. It is easiest to think of a liability as a debt, although this is not the only type of liability. Liabilities are any future obligations of the business. Examples include accounts payable (money owed to the pharmacy's suppliers), bank loans, and employee wages earned but not yet paid. Certain taxes can also accrue over time before they are due to be paid, and those are also a liability.

Stated plainly, assets can provide you with cash (e.g., if you were to collect accounts receivable or sell your property), while liabilities will require you to give up cash (e.g., such as when paying a supplier or bank loan).

*Equity* is the difference between the pharmacy's assets and liabilities. Think of a home purchased with a mortgage. The home's value (the asset) minus the loan balance (the liability) is the owner's equity in that property. In a similar way, a business's equity—all of its assets minus all of its liabilities—represents the net value of the business to its owner.

*Revenue*, sometimes referred to as *income* or *sales*, is a very broad term used to describe any money coming into the pharmacy for goods sold (e.g., prescriptions or OTC medications) or services delivered (e.g., medication therapy management, point-of-care testing.) It does not take into account anything that the pharmacy has paid or will need to pay (e.g., the cost of those items or employee wages) in order to provide those goods or services, as described in the paragraphs below.

*COGS* is the purchase cost of the medications and other items that the pharmacy sells, generally what the supplier charges for the specific inventory sold in a given period. To accurately calculate its COGS, a pharmacy must know its inventory on hand at the beginning and end of the period. COGS is then calculated as (beginning inventory + inventory acquired during the period − ending inventory).

*Gross profit* is revenue minus COGS and represents the direct contribution of a pharmacy's business operations to its overall profitability.

*Expenses* are the costs (current or future outlays of cash) required to operate the pharmacy. They may be supplier bills directly related to the items being sold such as prescriptions or OTC medications (see COGS above), people costs such as wages and benefits, or items of overhead such as rent and utilities.

*Profit*, or *net income*, is the amount of money earned after subtracting expenses from gross profit. In other words, this is the amount of money left over after taking into consideration employee salary, electricity, lease costs, insurance, security, inventory, and other expenses.

As an example of how these pieces fit together, if my new pharmacy had revenue of $35 000 last month and COGS was $28 000 with other expenses of $6000, my gross profit for the month was $7000 ($35 000 − $28 000 = $7000) and my profit, or net income, was $1000 ($7000 − $6000 = $1000).

## ■ FINANCIAL STATEMENTS

Financial statements are to a pharmacist what a global positioning system (GPS) is to a driver—they allow a community pharmacist to see where their pharmacy "has been" and where it is likely "to be going." Just like it may take some time to orient to a new GPS, it may take a community pharmacist new to financial statements some time to orient themselves to the report itself. Further complicating things is the fact that there is no one single format of these financial statements. Despite this, generally the information found on each of these statements and the statement's purpose are the same.

Several stakeholder types are interested in financial statements from your pharmacy. The most obvious stakeholder is the pharmacy manager. As described in the "Financial Analysis" section below, a pharmacy manager may use these financial statements to *benchmark*, that is, compare their pharmacy to others, in order to evaluate their pharmacy's performance. The statements allow pharmacy managers to make crucial decisions about many aspects of the business including staffing, inventory, and budgeting. A pharmacy owner or corporate leader, too, has an interest in these statements. Typically, the pharmacy manager may make quick, day-to-day decisions based on these reports, while owners and corporate leaders use this information to make long-term, strategic decisions about the direction of the organization, such as opening or permanently closing pharmacies, hiring and firing employees, and seeking new business loans.

Having familiarized yourselves with some of the basic financial terminology, you can now develop an understanding of the two most common financial statements: the Balance Sheet and Income Statement, often referred to as the Profit and Loss Statement, or simply, the P&L. A third statement required by GAAP, the cash flow statement, summarizes an organization's sources and uses of cash over the period of the income statement. While a more detailed discussion of this statement is beyond the scope of this chapter, we encourage the reader to learn more about this important statement and how it can be used as a tool for understanding and managing a pharmacy's operations.[2,3]

The *balance sheet* describes the financial position of the company by presenting the assets, liabilities, and equity of the business at a given point in time. The balance sheet is built on what's known as the basic accounting equation (Assets = Liabilities + Equity), and is typically presented in columnar format with assets on the left side of the page "in balance" with the total of liabilities and equity on the right side.

Assets and liabilities are generally segregated between current and noncurrent. Current assets are cash and those other assets likely to be turned into cash over the next 12 months, such as accounts receivable and inventory. Similarly, current liabilities are those obligations due within the next 12 months and might include a pharmacy's accounts payable as well as the next 12 months of loan payments (e.g., mortgage or equipment loans.) Reporting assets and liabilities in such a way allows the reader of the financial statements to assess the pharmacy's ability to meet its short-term obligations. An example of a basic balance sheet is shown in Figure 8-1.

The *income statement* presents the pharmacy's profit (or loss) over a given period of time by showing detailed line items of revenue and expense for the period. The statement begins by presenting the pharmacy's revenue from various sources and subtracting the cost of those items to arrive at a subtotal called gross profit. Additional expense categories are then presented line by line to arrive at net profit or net income, appropriately referred to as "the bottom line." However, depending on the complexity and structure of the business, certain expenses may be segregated from pharmacy operating expenses to present a more accurate calculation of income derived from business operations. In a larger organization this may be shown as Earnings before Interest, Taxes, Depreciation, and Amortization or EBITDA, but even a smaller community pharmacy will likely have some combination of those "nonoperating" expenses which are then subtracted to arrive at the enterprise's true "bottom line."

When a pharmacy's total sources of revenue exceed their total costs and expenses, it has generated a net profit. Costs and expenses in excess of total revenue result in a net loss. Net profits add to owner's equity; net losses reduce owner's equity. An example of a basic income statement is shown in Figure 8-2.

In summary, the balance sheet and the income statement present two very different, but equally important, types of information. The balance sheet presents a picture of the business's financial position at a point in time, generally the last day of the month or year. In contrast, the income statement presents the results of business operations over a period of time, such as the previous month, quarter, or year. However, the two statements are directly linked through the Owner's Equity account which is increased by the pharmacy's net income or decreased by its net loss.

In practice, the pharmacist or pharmacy manager may look to the income statement as the more valuable tool for evaluating short-term results and decision making while the owner or financial institution may find the balance sheet to be a more appropriate indicator of the pharmacy's overall health and longer-term prospects. However, both statements contain valuable

**Hohmeier Community Pharmacy**
**Balance Sheet**
**December 31, 2020**

| Assets | | Liabilities | |
|---|---|---|---|
| Current Assets | | Current Liabilities | |
| Cash | $10 000 | Accounts Payable | $120 000 |
| Accounts Receivable | 40 000 | Taxes Payable | 5 000 |
| Inventory | 180 000 | | 125 000 |
| | 230 000 | Non-current Liabilities | |
| Non-current Assets | | Bank Loan | 75 000 |
| Furniture & Fixtures | 20 000 | | |
| Equipment | 10 000 | **Total Liabilities** | **200 000** |
| Vehicles | 25 000 | | |
| | | **Owner's Equity** | **85 000** |
| **Total Assets** | **$285 000** | **Liabilities and Equity** | **$285 000** |

**Figure 8-1.** Sample balance sheet.

**Hohmeier Community Pharmacy**
**Income Statement**
**For the Twelve Months Ending December 31, 2020**

| | | |
|---|---:|---:|
| **Sales** | | |
| Prescriptions | $1 700 000 | |
| Over-the-counter medications | 25 000 | |
| Other merchandise | 275 000 | |
| Total sales | | $2 000 000 |
| Cost of goods sold | | 1 600 000 |
| **Gross profit** | | **400 000** |
| **Operating Expenses** | | |
| Salaries & benefits | 225 000 | |
| Insurance | 36 000 | |
| Rent | 24 000 | |
| Utilities | 18 000 | |
| Depreciation | 8 000 | |
| Vehicle expense | 8 000 | |
| Supplies | 7 000 | |
| Legal & accounting | 6 000 | |
| Total operating expenses | | 332 000 |
| **Income from Operations** | | **68 000** |
| Interest expense | | 5 000 |
| Income taxes | | 13 000 |
| **Net Income** | | **$50 000** |

**Figure 8-2.** Sample income statement.

information that should be used together in analyzing the pharmacy's performance.

# ▊ FINANCIAL STATEMENT ANALYSIS

Financial statement analysis allows the reader to use the pharmacy's financial statements to evaluate the health of the business currently and over time, and to make financial-related decisions. To facilitate comparisons and analysis, current period amounts are often shown alongside prior figures on the pharmacy's statements. In this guidebook, we will focus on three methods of analysis: horizontal analysis, vertical analysis, and ratio analysis.[2]

*Horizontal analysis* is the comparison of financial information over a series of reporting periods, while *vertical analysis* is the proportional analysis of a financial statement, where each line item in a financial statement is listed as a percentage of another item.

*Ratio analysis* is used to calculate the relative size of one number in relation to another. Horizontal, vertical, and ratio analysis can be performed on both the balance sheet and income statement.

*Horizontal analysis* documents the movement of the pharmacy's key financial statement line items from year to year or from month to month, to monitor progress or identify unexpected changes. Comparing results from period to period can help answer such questions as, "Are prescription sales growing as projected? Are payroll expenses increasing faster than revenue? Why have supply costs (e.g., prescription vials, bags, bottles) doubled in the third quarter?" On the balance sheet, a trend of decreasing cash and increasing accounts receivable might indicate a slowing of patient prescription volume or delayed payment from third-party payers that should be addressed.

*Vertical analysis* is the review of financial statement line items expressed as a percentage of another single line item—most often total assets on the balance sheet and revenue on the income statement.

Those percentages can be compared to the pharmacy's prior results, to budgets and plans, or to similar-sized operations within the industry, referred to as benchmarking. For example, a pharmacy that spends 3% of its revenue on advertising and promotion when the industry average is 1% may find it can reduce its spending in that area. And, as the largest expense item on the income statement, it can be useful to benchmark salaries and benefits expenses against industry averages to evaluate a pharmacy's staffing efficiency.

Lastly, *ratio analysis* is the comparison of one financial statement line item to another. Much like the results of vertical analysis, a pharmacy's ratios should be compared to its own prior results and budgets, as well as to industry benchmarks when available. Ratios can be calculated on the balance sheet, the income statement, or across both statements. Important profitability ratios include *gross profit margin* (gross profit divided by total sales), *net profit margin* (net profit divided by total sales), and *break-even* calculations. Liquidity ratios such as the *current ratio* (all current assets divided by all current liabilities) and *quick ratio* (only *liquid* current assets such as cash and accounts receivable divided by all current liabilities) help to assess the pharmacy's health and ability to meet its operating obligations. *Debt-to-equity* and *debt service coverage* (annual operating income divided by annual loan payments) are leverage ratios that can indicate the pharmacy's reliance on debt and its ability to repay those loans.

While a more in-depth discussion of financial statement analysis is beyond the scope of this chapter, a simple internet search will help you understand these and many other tools available to help evaluate and guide your pharmacy operations.

## RISK MANAGEMENT

Financial *risk* in business generally refers to the possibility of falling short on your projected profit, or in some cases, having losses. All businesses inherently have risks as part of their operations. Risk can be seen in the form of lower-than-expected prescription volume, fluctuations in inventory costs, or declining reimbursement rates from third-party payers. On a larger scale, risk can also be seen when there is economic downturn, federal or state policy changes, or market disruptors (e.g., Amazon®, mail order pharmacy, COVID-19 pandemic). For example, during the Great Recession (2007–2010) small business failures increased by 40%.[4] Although risk cannot ever completely be avoided, there are ways to mitigate risk.

Financial Risks may include:

- Price (e.g., inventory purchasing costs, prescription backorders)
- Liquidity (e.g., cash flow, cash on hand)
- Credit (e.g., loan default, credit downgrade)

Each pharmacy's approach to risk will be different because the risk is unique to that pharmacy's characteristics. These factors which impact risk may include location, patient population, payer-mix (e.g., third-party payers contracted with the pharmacy), and services offered, to name a few. However, there are comprehensive ways for a pharmacist to systematically uncover their pharmacy's risk and make plans to limit that risk. One popular strategy is known as enterprise risk management (ERM).[5]

The use of ERM in community pharmacy varies widely, but general ERM principles should apply to most community pharmacies. It is not a single strategy to assess and mitigate risk, but a set of strategies and analytical tools from which a business may choose. ERM usually involves either statistical or structural modeling involving the use of both available data (e.g., profit, loss, debt) and expert opinion (e.g., future risk, relationships between data, past experience). In all cases, ERM is just a guess, but because of its use of both experts and mathematical modeling, it makes for an educated guess.

A community pharmacist would likely never be asked to select an ERM approach; however, they may be asked to apply specific ERM reports to their pharmacy and compare against benchmarks or internal metrics. For example, a common ERM metric seen in community pharmacy is EBITDA. This number approximates cash flow for the business and is useful in understanding current pharmacy operations and may also be used to *valuate* (i.e., appraise or estimate the value, or selling price, of a community pharmacy.)

Although risk can never be eliminated, a pharmacist should attempt to plan strategically around risk and identify mechanisms to mitigate it. As with financial analysis, there are standards and best practices which can be used to approach risk to your pharmacy. Having a foundational knowledge of risk and risk mitigation strategies will allow you to work with a professional with expertise in risk management (e.g., business manager consultant, consultancy firm, or lawyer) to outline a plan that is right for you and your pharmacy.

## ■ CHAPTER APPLICATIONS

1. At the beginning of this chapter "Setting the Scene," you were promoted to co-manager of a pharmacy, but had little experience with financial reporting. What are the two primary reports you would expect to use to help you assess the financial and operational performance of the pharmacy and how are they related?

2. The pharmacy just underwent a major remodel over the past 6 months. Which section(s) of the balance sheet would this remodel likely impact?

3. Your pharmacy's beginning inventory was $250 000. Using the financial statements shown in Figures 8-1 and 8-2 and the formula for determining COGS, what was the amount of inventory purchased over the reporting period?

4. Based on the reimbursement amounts you were familiar with when dispensing medications in the workflow, you had assumed that the pharmacy was "making money hand over fist." However, when analyzing the pharmacy reports you realized there were many expenses you had not considered which greatly reduced that number. What are the two terms for the line items on the income statement which correspond to your assessments?

5. Using the financial statements shown in Figures 8-1 and 8-2, calculate the pharmacy's Current Ratio, Quick Ratio, and Gross Profit Percentage. What do these metrics tell us about the pharmacy's operations?[6]

6. Let's say that last year, a nationwide economic recession has placed additional pressures on the pharmacy organization. As part of an annual strategic planning exercise, you are asked to review the pharmacy's cash flow and compare it to the organization's historical benchmarks to better understand overall pharmacy operations and how the pharmacy has withstood the recession. What type of planning is this exercise called? And, what type of metric could be used in this planning exercise?

## REFERENCES

1. American Association of Colleges of Pharmacy. Guidance for the Accreditation Standards and Key Elements for the Professional Program in Pharmacy Leading to the Doctor of Pharmacy Degree. Published February 2, 2015. Accessed May 26, 2021. https://www.acpe-accredit.org/pdf/GuidanceforStandards2016FINAL.pdf

2. Chisholm-Burns MA, Vaillancourt AM, Shepherd M. *Pharmacy Management, Leadership, Marketing, and Finance*. 1st ed. Sudbury, MA: Jones & Bartlett Publishers; 2011.

3. Zgarrick DP, Alston GL. *Pharmacy Management: Essentials for All Practice Settings*. 5th ed. Sudbury, MA: Jones & Bartlett Publishers; 2020.

4. Harner MM. Mitigating financial risk for small business entrepreneurs. *Ohio St. Entrepren. Bus. LJ*. 2011; 6:469.

5. Casualty Actuarial Society. Enterprise Risk Management Committee. Overview of Enterprise Risk Management. Published May, 2003. Accessed May 26, 2021. https://erm.ncsu.edu/az/erm/i/chan/m-articles/documents/CasualtyActuarialSocietyOverviewofERM.pdf

6. 2019 NCPA Digest. The State of Retail Pharmacy: Independent Pharmacy Economics Stabilize—But Dropping, Owner Salaries Are (as referenced in drugchannels.net article). Drugchannels. Published December 3, 2019. Accessed May 26, 2021. https://www.drugchannels.net/2019/12/the-state-of-retail-pharmacy.html

# 9

# PAYMENT MODELS AND METHODS

*Jay Bueche, RPh, and Rannon Ching, PharmD*

---

## ▨ LEARNING OBJECTIVES

1. Explain how healthcare benefits are administered in the United States.
2. Differentiate the types of healthcare benefits and payers that pharmacists can contract with for payment of products and services.
3. Define the types of pharmacy benefit network structures.
4. Describe how financial terms of pharmacy benefit contracts are structured.

## ■ SETTING THE SCENE

After graduating and working as a staff pharmacist for 2 years, you decide to take the plunge into ownership. Your new pharmacy seems very successful offering a wide range of services in addition to accepting all major third-party plans. After you dig into the books, it appears the previous owner was not charging or was undercharging for services and third-party profit dropped by 10% each of the last 2 years. A few weeks later, you receive a notice that the pharmacy owes $20 000 to a major Medicare plan for something called DIR fees. Quickly, you realize understanding how to get paid is the key to survival for your pharmacy.

In 2019, 95% of all prescriptions purchased in the United States were paid or processed through a third-party payer.[1] Understanding how to manage and maximize third-party revenue is now an essential role of all pharmacists and pharmacy technicians—not just owners and managers. Additionally, profit from prescription revenue will likely shrink in the future as new competitors enter the marketplace, politicians and the public continue to scrutinize the cost of prescription drugs and technology and convenience force change within the pharmacy marketplace.

The U.S. healthcare payment model is highly complex with multiple benefit structures, payers, and billing formats. As the role of the pharmacist in patient care services grows, getting paid will depend on understanding each of these components.

## ■ BENEFIT STRUCTURES

The U.S. healthcare payment system is a collection of different benefit structures. For instance, a dental benefit pays for services at the dentist, the medical benefit covers doctor and hospital visits and the pharmacy benefit offsets costs of prescription drugs. Pharmacies frequently bill claims under both the prescription and medical benefit.

Within each benefit structure there is also a *plan design*. Elements of a plan design include the premium, deductible, list of covered services, cost-sharing amounts and, in the instance of the pharmacy benefit, the formulary.

- *Premiums* are routine payments made to an insurance plan. For instance, an employee may pay a monthly premium of $200 to participate in the company-sponsored health coverage.
- *Deductibles* are the amount paid by the *insured* (the individual covered by the insurance plan) out-of-pocket before the plan begins to cover, or pay, for a portion of the services.
- *Covered services* are the services in which some or all of the cost is paid by the plan.
- *Cost-sharing* is the amount paid by the insured for a covered service. Cost-sharing is sometimes divided into *copayments* (e.g., copays) and *coinsurance*. *Copayments* are standard flat dollar amounts. For instance, an emergency room visit under a plan may have a $200 copay. *Coinsurance* amounts are typically a percentage of the cost of the service. For example, the emergency room visit cost $1800, and the *coinsurance* amount is 10%, so the insured would pay $180.
- The *formulary* is the list of medications covered by the plan. Not all medications may be covered (i.e., some are non-formulary), but those that are, are typically divided into *tiers*. Each tier will have separate cost-sharing levels. For instance, "tier one" is often inexpensive generics and may have low cost-sharing (e.g., $5 copay) requirements. Higher tiers will include more expensive medications and have a greater level of cost-sharing (e.g., $50 copay).

## ■ PAYERS

### Commercial Insurance

Commercial insurance refers to private plans paid for by individuals, employers, unions, or other organizations. While commercial plans often fall under federal or state regulations, the types of benefits offered and the plan design vary widely. Commercial plans can account for a large portion of a pharmacy's prescription revenue, so understanding these contracts and benefits is important.

## Medicaid

Medicaid is a program providing coverage for eligible low-income adults, pregnant women, and children. Eligibility varies from state to stage but to qualify individuals must meet certain income or other resource criteria. Medicaid is a program that is jointly funded by federal and state governments but administered by States. Prescription drug coverage is optional, but as of 2018, was covered by all 50 States plus the District of Columbia.[2]

## Medicare

Medicare is a federally funded healthcare benefit for individuals over the age of 65 and certain people with disabilities regardless of age.[3] Medicare has several benefits, some of which are optional, including hospital, long-term care, medical insurance, and prescription drugs.

## ◼ ALTERNATE PAYMENT METHODS

### Discount Cards

Discount cards are widely available and may offer patients the ability to pay less than the pharmacy's cash or usual and customary (U&C) price. Discount card rates are included in contracts with pharmacy benefit managers (PBMs), but patients are responsible for paying the entire discounted portion of the medication (i.e., there is no payer to cover any of the cost) plus an administrative fee paid back to the PBM. Discount cards are marketed by brokers such as GoodRx®, Singlecare®, Retailmenot®, Blink® to name a few. These discount cards are available through the company website, phone application, mail-out cards, or available at the pharmacy.

### Copay Assistance Cards and Patient Assistance Programs

Prescription manufacturers may offer copay cards and patient assistance programs to help patients afford higher cost, usually branded medications. Copay cards are funded by manufacturers and can be used to lower a patient's insurance cost-sharing amount by paying a remittance to the pharmacy. These copay cards may be available at the pharmacy, provided to the patient from their physician's office, or obtained from the manufacturer website. Patient assistance programs are available for certain medications and these applications may be accessed on the manufacturer's website. Pharmacies or physician office personnel may help patients access these applications for assistance, and patient eligibility is usually based on their annual income. Each manufacturer has different eligibility criteria and application processes for medication assistance. These types of programs are generally not available to individuals enrolled in government benefits (e.g., Medicare, Medicaid, and so on) but this will vary based upon manufacturer guidelines.

### Cash-Based Products and Services

Cash-based services are a fast growing area within pharmacy and healthcare. Just like it sounds, cash-based (also called out-of-pocket) means that there is a flat fee that is paid by the patient to receive the product or service. Purchasing an item from a retail store or a ticket to an amusement park is the common example of the cash-based model. The beauty of this model is that the payment process becomes extremely simple. If a patient wants to utilize your pharmacy's service or product, they pay a fee directly to the pharmacy. No submitting to insurance, discount cards, audits, rejected claims, or prior authorizations.

There are community pharmacies that do not accept insurance for prescriptions and dispense medications at competitive out-of-pocket prices, while maintaining profitable margins. Benefits of this model include being able to offer cheap out-of-pocket costs for generic medications lower than typical insurance copays, and profitability is not in the hands of MAC lists (maximum allowable costs), generic effective rates (GER), or middlemen. The downside of this model is that they can usually only offer generic products, because the high cost of brand name drugs are not practical for most patients without insurance.

Point-of-care testing (POCT) is a great opportunity for cash-based services. Examples of CLIA-waived POCT include COVID-19 rapid testing, rapid flu, rapid strep, blood glucose, cholesterol panels, and A1C levels. These tests may be covered by insurance, but billing delays may impact patients who are in need of timely testing and results. This idea of payment for convenience is one of the key factors for deciding whether a service or product can be cash-based. The ease and convenience of being able to conduct timely POCT services for patients at the local pharmacy on nights, weekends, and on a walk-in basis is needed and appealing.

Determining prices for cash-based services is a mixture of art and science. Profitability, market competition, ease of access, surrounding socioeconomic landscapes, supply, and demand are factors in pricing decisions.

## ■ NETWORK STRUCTURES

Health plans and PBMs contract with pharmacies to dispense medications and provide services. Pharmacies contracted with the plan are considered *in-network* (i.e., pharmacies within the same payer network) while all others are *out-of-network*.

There are several types of network structures in which pharmacies may participate. *Broad* networks include any pharmacy willing to contract with the plan while *limited* or *narrow* networks include a smaller subset. *Preferred* networks typically include all pharmacies, but patient cost-sharing amounts may be less at *preferred pharmacies*. Preferred pharmacy networks are common in Medicare and other government programs required to allow all pharmacies to participate (i.e., "any willing pharmacy").

To participate in narrow or preferred networks, pharmacies must be willing to accept a lower reimbursement rate. In return, pharmacies should be able to gain additional patients (i.e., market share). Making the decision to participate in these networks must be carefully evaluated by community pharmacies in terms of lost prescription revenue, but also in additional foot traffic and non-pharmacy sales.

## ■ THIRD-PARTY CONTRACTING

While large chains typically contract directly, independent pharmacies and small chains typically work with a Pharmacy Services Administration Organization (PSAO) for the majority of their contracts. There are a handful of independent PSAOs, but each of the large wholesalers also operate a PSAO.

While immunizations and nondispensing services are a growing part of the pharmacy business, most revenue is still generated by dispensing traditional medications. Contracts with PBMs can be complex legal documents and should be reviewed by legal professionals; however, the reimbursement or "rate" portion of the contract will require careful financial review by the business owner. To be profitable, a pharmacy must ensure third-party payments and other revenue exceeds the cost of procuring product plus all expenses (e.g., payroll, rent, and utilities).

## ■ BASICS OF PHARMACY CLAIM PROCESSING

Virtually every PBM agreement requires electronic claims processing (i.e., adjudication) through the most current National Council of Prescription Drug Plan (NCPDP) standard. Adjudication typically occurs in real time (less than a second) via an electronic mechanism called a "switch" and allows the PBM and pharmacy, by submitting claim information in standard fields and segments (i.e., patient, prescriber, product, claim, etc.). The pharmacy will instantly receive copay and reimbursement details after claim adjudication. Pharmacy claim processing is in real time, opposed to medical claim processing where payment details may take days to weeks to be communicated to the medical office.

The pharmacy's dispensing system will display the reimbursement for each claim. The payment calculation can involve multiple fields including sales tax values and amounts paid by other payers using a process called the *coordination of benefits*. For a claim involving only one third-party payer, 4 fields can be used to calculate the pharmacy's reimbursement: *ingredient cost paid*, *dispensing fee paid*, *patient pay amount*, and *total amount paid*. Note each dispensing application might have different names or terminology, but the standard NCPDP names are used below.

- *Ingredient cost paid*: Contractual amount due to pharmacy to cover the cost of the dispensed product.
- *Dispensing fee paid*: Contractual dispensing fee amount paid to the pharmacy.
- *Patient pay amount*: The total amount due by the patient, also known as the copay.
- *Total amount paid*: Amount owed to the pharmacy by the PBM.

## Brand Reimbursement

Payment for brand medications is tied to a public pricing benchmark—most commonly *average wholesale price* (AWP), plus a dispensing fee. AWP is reported by the drug manufacturer and theoretically represents the amount paid by a pharmacy to buy a product from a wholesaler. This benchmark is commonly used to calculate pharmacy reimbursements in third-party contracts. Contracts typically set reimbursement as a discount off AWP (e.g., AWP—17%).

## Generic Reimbursement

The most common reimbursement mechanism for generic medications is MAC. Generally, PBMs have wide latitude on which medications will have an MAC and what that reimbursement will be. Contracts typically allow pharmacies to challenge the MAC price if it is too low through a *MAC Appeals* process.

Larger chains often have *effective rate* agreements for generic medications, where a benchmark is set for a guaranteed average reimbursement. While effective rate contracts afford pharmacies a more predictable payment structure for generics, complex analytics are also required to ensure appropriate reimbursement is received. Effective rates can increase reimbursement if found to be below the benchmark; however, the reverse is also true. Reimbursements found to be over the benchmark could be recouped from the pharmacy due to following the benchmark average.

It is important to understand that the profit is the difference between what the pharmacy paid for the drug and the reimbursement received. *Wholesale acquisition cost* (WAC) is reported by the drug manufacturer and is supposed to represent the price paid by a drug wholesaler for the product. This benchmark is commonly used by pharmacies when contracting with drug wholesalers. Therefore, you would ideally want the WAC to be significantly lower than the AWP or MAC.

## ■ GETTING PAID BY MEDICARE

Medicare is the federal health insurance plan providing health coverage for people ages 65 and older, certain younger people with disabilities, and those with end-stage renal disease.[3] Medicare is managed by the Centers for Medicare and Medicaid Services (CMS). There are 3 different benefits within Medicare offering coverage for different services:

- Medicare Part A (Hospital Insurance): Covers inpatient hospital stays, care in a skilled nursing facility, hospice care, and some home healthcare
- Medicare Part B (Medical Insurance): Covers certain doctors' services, outpatient care, medical supplies (e.g., durable medical equipment [DME]), and preventive services
- Medicare Part D (Prescription Drug Coverage): Helps cover the cost of prescription drugs (including some recommended shots or vaccines)[3]

There are 2 different options for Medicare coverage, which include Original Medicare and Medicare

Advantage. Original Medicare includes Part A and Medicare Part B, with the option to add a separate Part D for drug costs. In community pharmacies, we primarily deal with Part D plans and a select number of services, products and medications covered under Part B.

## How to Join Medicare

There are several opportunities for patients to either sign up for Medicare or change their current benefits. Patients will often ask pharmacy staff questions regarding switching plans or prescription coverage, so it is important to have a baseline knowledge to help patients with Medicare plan selection. The main 3 opportunities for patients to join, switch, or drop Medicare plans include:

- Initial Enrollment Period:
  - Patients become eligible for Medicare
  - 7-month period starting 3 months before the age of 65, the month people turn 65, and the following 3 months after turning 65
- Open Enrollment Period
  - Each year between October 15 and December 7
  - Coverage starting January 1
- Medicare Advantage Open Enrollment Period
  - Each year from January 1 to March 31

## Structure of Medicare Part D Plans

Like commercial plans, there are many differences between Medicare Part D Plans. Patients can choose between various Medicare plans, plan types, and coverages. Medicare Part D premiums, which is the cost that the patient must pay for that plan's coverage each month, vary by plan with higher-income consumers possibly paying more. Generally, higher premiums translate to a bigger formulary of covered drugs, lower or no deductibles, and potentially lower copay tier structures. That is not always the case, but the thought is that higher monthly premiums put more money in the collective pot to be distributed to the insured members. Patients should look at total plan costs for the year, not just the plan premium when selecting a standalone Medicare Part D plan. It is possible for the Part D plan with a high

premium to actually be the cheapest for some patients due to the variations in formularies, cost-sharing and deductibles. Most Part D plans are structured in a phased design, which includes the deductible, initial coverage, coverage gap, and catastrophic phase. These phases reset at the beginning of each plan year—which is January 1 for Medicare.

- *Deductible Phase*: The patient will pay copays for 100% of services, up to a certain amount, before the Medicare drug plan starts to pay its share. Deductibles vary between plans, but none of the plans can have a deductible larger than the limit that CMS sets for each year. Some plans do not have deductibles, so those patients would go straight into the initial coverage phase.
- *Initial Coverage Phase*: The drug plan begins to cover a portion of drug costs, and patients would begin to pay copays in accordance to their drug formulary and tier structure, which differs with each plan. The initial coverage phase lasts until the drug plan contributes a set amount toward the patient's drug costs, then it progresses into the coverage gap phase.
- *Coverage Gap Phase*: The coverage gap phase (often called the "donut hole") is when cost-sharing may increase for some medications. Once the patient has paid a certain dollar amount for copays during this period, they will enter the final phase of catastrophic coverage.
- *Catastrophic Coverage Phase*: Once patients have paid a certain dollar amount out-of-pocket, they will get through the coverage gap and into the catastrophic coverage phase. This phase makes sure that patients' copays or coinsurance are small amounts for the rest of the year.

Some patients may qualify for *Extra Help* depending on income and financial resources or assets. Extra Help can pay for or reduce premiums and cost-sharing for eligible patients.

## What to Do When a Patient's Copays Increase?

Most community pharmacists have heard the question, "Why is my copay so high?" or "My copay is supposed to be lower than this!" There are a few things pharmacists can do to investigate why there are changes to a copay.

The first thing to do is to determine which benefit stage the patient is in. The *benefit stage qualifier code* corresponds to which insurance phase a patient is in. This will answer where the copay is going or being applied to.

Benefit Stage Qualifier Code:

- 01: Deductible Phase
- 02: Initial Benefit Phase
- 03: Coverage Gap Phase
- 04: Catastrophic Phase

Most pharmacy software can show you if the copay is being applied toward a deductible, which means the patient is in the deductible phase of their plan. Remember that the deductible phase means the patient is responsible for 100% of the drug cost, until they meet the out-of-pocket requirement for their specific plan. This is why it is important to know when plans reset their deductible, and ask the patient if their plan has renewed or changed. Sometimes, if a patient is close to meeting their deductible, you'll see a portion of the copay going to the deductible, while the rest of the copay is following the tier structure of the initial benefit stage.

Example: A patient has $25 left on their deductible, and their copay is $75. Your computer system shows that $25 of the copay is being applied to the deductible, and the other $50 is the drug price taking into account the initial coverage copay tiers.

If a patient is in the coverage gap phase, you can inform the patient that they're in the donut hole and explain that they will have to pay a higher percentage of their medications, unless they pay enough out-of-pocket costs to get out of the donut hole.

## Pharmacy Direct and Indirect Remuneration (DIR)

Medicare Part D has a highly complex financial structure that involves funding by the Federal Government, Medicare enrollees and Part D plans. Medicare tracks all patient and plan expenses and payments, and shares risks with Part D plans. Rebates paid to Part D plans are tracked as *Direct and Indirect Remuneration* (DIR).[4] The largest portion of DIR is manufacturer rebates; however, pharmacy rebates paid to plans have grown substantially in recent years. In fact, CMS noted that pharmacy DIR grew by 45,000% between 2010 and 2017.[5]

Pharmacy DIR payment amounts are set contractually and are often determined based on the pharmacy's "performance" according to plan determined criteria. The measurements for these programs can be arbitrary (e.g., generic dispensing rate) but are often based on *Medicare Star Ratings* such as medication adherence and medication therapy management (MTM) completion rates. See Chapter 10, "Quality Metrics" for additional information about DIR fees and mitigating their effect.

## Medicare Star Rating Measurements

Medicare Star Ratings are published by CMS for the purpose of measuring the quality of service and health outcomes delivered by Medicare plans. For 2021, there are 32 Star measures for Medicare Advantage and up to 14 for standalone Medicare Part D plans.[6]

Medication adherence is measured based on a calculation called proportion of days covered (PDC). In essence, PDC reflects the percentage of time (i.e., days in a calendar year) a patient has enough medication available. To calculate PDC, take the total number of days covered by refills in a measurement period and divide by the number of days between the first fill and the end of the measurement period. Medicare deems a patient to be compliant with a PDC of 80% or greater. Medicare currently measures 3 classes of patient populations for adherence: individuals taking a statin, renin-angiotensin system agonist or oral diabetic medication (and not using insulin).[7] Typically, plans and pharmacies are measured based on the number of patients in a particular category who are adherent. For instance, if a pharmacy has 100 patients taking a statin and 85 are adherent, then the adherence measure would be 85%.

Another pharmacy measure is the MTM completion rate. For this measure, the focus is completion of comprehensive medication reviews (CMR). CMS sets criteria for patients eligible for MTM—typically those with more than 1 chronic condition, on multiple mediations and total cost of medications over a set amount. A CMR involves an interactive medication review or consultation between a patient and the pharmacist. Pharmacists review the patient's prescription and nonprescription medications they take for adverse events, duplications, omissions, interactions, and evaluate appropriate medication use including adherence. The measure is calculated based on the percentage of eligible patients who have a completed CMR.[8]

## Medicare Part B and Pharmacy

Medicare Part B pays for services traditionally delivered by outpatient medical providers; however, pharmacies can still bill and get paid for some services through Part B. The most common services billed under Medicare Part B are immunizations, diabetes testing supplies, DME, some nebulized medications, and other various medical services (e.g., POCT).

To bill Medicare Part B, pharmacies must enroll with Medicare and receive a Provider Transaction Access Number (PTAN). Part B claims are billed as a medical benefit, so most pharmacies utilize a third-party processor through their existing pharmacy software. Immunizations for influenza and pneumonia are the most commonly billed items through Medicare Part B in a pharmacy setting.

## ▊ GETTING PAID BY MEDICAID

The Medicaid program is separately administered by each state government under the oversight of CMS. State Medicaid programs can take a variety of forms. Traditionally, Medicaid benefits were completely administered by state governments under *Fee-For-Service* (FFS) arrangements, meaning that providers billed for, and were paid for, each individual service provided.[9] Some states use a payment model called *managed care* in which private *Managed Care Organizations* (MCOs), or health plans, contract with the state Medicaid to administer benefits.

To participate in a state's Medicaid program, pharmacists often must contract, or apply, to participate. If all or part of the program is administered under managed care, the pharmacy must also contract with each individual MCO. A separate enrollment is often required for heavy durable medical equipment (DME; e.g., walkers, wheelchairs, and hospital beds).

## Value-Based Purchasing (VBP)

*Value-based purchasing* (VBP), or contracting arrangements, have evolved from federal legislation to encourage provider accountability and reward performance and quality. While hospitals and physicians were the initial focus of VBP, pharmacies are slowly being included in performance contracts. Some of these contracts can be as simple as pharmacies providing new services such as administration of medications or vaccines, MTM or disease state education. See Chapter 11, "Clinical and Value-Based Services" for additional services that could be provided. Other arrangements involve pharmacies taking some degree of financial risk. Risk models include *upside* and *downside* risk. In downside risk arrangements, the health plan and provider share the savings or loss associated with patient care. If the plan is profitable, then the provider benefits, but if the plan loses money, then the provider shares in the loss.

Pharmacies typically participate in *upside* risk or "shared savings" arrangements. This type of contract may involve standard reimbursement for medication dispensing and additional payments if certain performance thresholds are met. For instance, a pharmacy may receive a quality bonus if a certain percentage of patients are adherent to a medication. While there is not a chance of direct loss, the pharmacy may have to dedicate resources to achieve the target performance. It is important to carefully evaluate what effort and resources are necessary to achieve the bonus payout before committing to a value-based contract.

# 340B

## Overview

The 340B Drug Pricing Program was created in 1992 by an act of Congress and is named after the authorizing section of the Public Health Services Act. The 340B program allows certain clinics and health systems (i.e., 340B-covered entities) to obtain medication at a substantially reduced price to offset costs associated with providing uncompensated care. Only outpatient services are eligible for 340B. Medicaid prescriptions are generally excluded from 340B as States receive rebates from manufacturers which would result in a "duplicate discount."

## Contract Pharmacies

340B-covered entities can partner with contract community pharmacies to provide medication services to their patients and to obtain an additional source of revenue. By participating as a contract pharmacy, there is an opportunity to gain new patients and additional profit from 340B dispensing fees. Unlike traditional benefits where pharmacies receive payment for the cost of the medication and a dispensing fee, 340B involves a larger dispensing fee and replenishment of product.

Covered entities without in-house community pharmacies often contract with outside pharmacies to dispense medications on their behalf. Contract pharmacies dispense medications from their own stock and in return receive a dispensing fee typically ranging between $8 and $15 (as compared to a $0-2 dispensing fee for traditional PBM contracts) plus replenished product.[10]

Even if a 340B-covered entity does not use an outside pharmacy to dispense medications, prescriptions for a qualified visit may still be 340B eligible. In these instances, covered entities may be entitled to receive revenue for eligible "third-party" prescriptions dispensed at contract pharmacies. In return, pharmacies receive products and an enhanced dispensing fee.

Under 340B, a product is not received by the pharmacy until a full package size threshold is reached. For example, if a medication comes in a bottle of 100 tablets and is dispensed in 30 count increments, it would take 4 fills to be replenished. As such, pharmacies may be in a "negative cash flow" meaning that product was initially purchased and dispensed well before replenishment occurred. Due to the challenges of accounting for and managing a 340B program, it is important that pharmacy owners or leaders carefully evaluate the financial impact and all relevant factors (e.g., wholesaler rebates, DIR) prior to becoming a 340B contract pharmacy.

# CHAPTER APPLICATIONS

1. MS is a 72-year-old female that has prescription insurance through a Medicare plan. She comes into the pharmacy to pick up her monthly prescription of Xarelto 20 mg, and is shocked at the copay which is $103.89. She emphatically tells you that the price is incorrect because her usual copay is $45. Being the savvy provider that you are, you suspect that there is a reason for the price increase. The full cost of the medication is $415.59 for a 30-day supply. Which of the following could account for the price increase? Select all that would apply:
   A. Patient is in Benefit Stage Qualifier 01.
   B. Patient is in Benefit Stage Qualifier 02.
   C. Patient is in Benefit Stage Qualifier 03.
   D. Patient is in Benefit Stage Qualifier 04.
2. ES is a 52-year-old male that has commercial prescription insurance. He comes to the pharmacy to pick up a new medication for Myrbetriq 25 mg. Because the medication is a brand name, his insurance requires the patient to pay a 25% coinsurance charge for a 30-day supply. If the medication cost is $398.00 for a 30-day supply, how much will the copay be for ES?
   A. $55.00
   B. $298.50
   C. $398.00
   D. $99.50
3. The pharmacy owner is reviewing a claim to ensure proper payment was received. The rate

section of the contract for ACME PBM states the pharmacy is to be reimbursed as follows:

Brands: AWP-18% +$0.50 Dispensing Fee
Generics: MAC + $0.50

Prescription # 42865
Product Dispensed: Invokana 300 mg
Dispensed quantity: #30
Published Average Wholesale Price per tablet: $22

Below are the pricing fields in the pharmacy dispensing system. Was the pharmacy reimbursed correctly?

Ingredient Cost Paid: $541.20
Dispensing Fee: $0.50
Patient Pay Amount: $80
Total Amount Paid: $461.70

4. The pharmacy receives a Medicare Part D contract with a "performance" section. The pharmacy's reimbursement will be AWP-15% +$0.50 less a DIR fee based on the adherence of their patient population based on the schedule below:

80% or less of patients are adherent to statin therapy for the contract period, DIR fee of 7% of AWP for each prescription

80.1–90% of patients are adherent to statin therapy for the contract period, DIR fee of 4% of AWP for each prescription

90.1% or greater of patients are adherent to statin therapy for the contract period, DIR fee of 0% of AWP for each prescription

The contract period is the upcoming calendar year.

a. What would the pharmacy need to know to be able to develop an action plan to address patient adherence?

b. What action(s) might the pharmacy want to take to improve patient adherence?

## REFERENCES

1. Number of Retail Prescription Drugs Filled at Pharmacies by Payer (Timeframe 2019). KFF website: Accessed January 30, 2021. https://www.kff.org/health-costs/state-indicator/total-retail-rx-drugs/?dataView=1&currentTimeframe=0&sortModel=%7B%22colId%22:%22Location%22,%22sort%22:%22asc%22%7D

2. Medicaid Prescription Drug Benefits: Key Facts. KFF website. Published May 1, 2019. Accessed May 26, 2021. https://www.kff.org/medicaid/fact-sheet/medicaids-prescription-drug-benefit-key-facts/

3. Medicare and Medicaid Basics, Medicare Learning Network, United States Center for Medicare & Medicaid Services, July 2018, ICN 909330.

4. Medicare Part D—Direct and Indirect Remuneration (DIR) Fact Sheet. United States Center for Medicare and Medicaid Services. Published January 19, 2017. Accessed January 30, 2021. https://www.cms.gov/newsroom/fact-sheets/medicare-part-d-direct-and-indirect-remuneration-dir

5. Proposed Rule: Modernizing Part D and Medicare Advantage to Lower Drug Prices and Reduce Out-of-Pocket Expenses (CMS-4180-P). United States Center for Medicare and Medicaid Services. Published November 2018. Accessed February 7, 2021. https://www.federalregister.gov/documents/2018/11/30/2018-25945/modernizing-part-d-and-medicare-advantage-to-lower-drug-prices-and-reduce-out-of-pocket-expenses

6. Fact Sheet—2021 Part C and Part D Star Ratings. United States Center for Medicare and Medicaid Services. Published October 13, 2020. Accessed February 7, 2021. https://www.cms.gov/files/document/2021starratings factsheet-10-13-2020.pdf

7. Schwartz L, Reese D, Rogers A. Quality Measures. America's Pharmacist. Alexandria, VA: National Community Pharmacists Association; June 2014.

8. Pattah V. MTM and the CMR Completion Rate: What Community Pharmacists Need to Know. Pharmacy Quality Measures. America's Pharmacist. Alexandria, VA: National Community Pharmacists Association; June 2015.

9. Medicaid Delivery System and Payment Reform: A Guide to Key Terms and Concepts, Kaiser Family Foundation. Published June 22, 2015. Accessed January 30, 2021. https://www.kff.org/medicaid/fact-sheet/medicaid-delivery-system-and-payment-reform-a-guide-to-key-terms-and-concepts/

10. Medicare Payment Advisory Committee. Overview of the 340B Drug Pricing Program: Report to Congress. Published May 2015. Accessed May 26, 2021. http://www.medpac.gov/docs/default-source/reports/may-2015-report-to-the-congress-overview-of-the-340b-drug-pricing-program.pdf?sfvrsn=0#:~:text=vii-,executive%20summary,than%20vaccines)%20from%20drug%20manufacturers

# 10

# QUALITY METRICS

*Chelsea P. Renfro, PharmD, James Cong, PharmD, and Benjamin Y. Urick, PharmD*

---

## ▓ LEARNING OBJECTIVES

1. Describe quality concepts in performance-based payment models.
2. Explain current performance-based issues facing community pharmacies.
3. Apply strategies to improve performance scores in the community pharmacy setting.

## ■ SETTING THE SCENE

Imagine taking your car to the mechanic because it won't start. He takes a look at it, and says that you need a new alternator. He also mentions that while he was looking at your car he noticed you needed a new air filter and your brake fluid changed. When you get the bill, you notice you were charged a fee for each item replaced as well as the mechanic's time. You need your car to be able to get to school and work, so you pay the bill. This type of transaction is how a fee-for-service healthcare model works.

Now imagine getting in your car several days later to head to school, and it won't start again. You remember that your mechanic provides a warranty on his work. You go back to the same mechanic, who then reassesses your car and realizes that the alternator was faulty and replaces it. Because the part is covered by the warranty, he doesn't charge you for the new alternator or his time. This payment is based on the quality of the services provided and is therefore only paid based on the initial services provided, which had an agreed upon quality of service (i.e., the warranty). This is similar to how a value-based care model works. Throughout this chapter, you will learn how the United States' healthcare system has shifted toward a value-based care model and the impact this has had on community pharmacy.

## ■ INTRODUCTION

Excessive spending and insufficient quality have driven calls for healthcare reform in the United States. As of 2019, 17.7% of the U.S. gross domestic product was spent on healthcare, far exceeding spending by other industrialized nations.[1] Additionally, reports comparing the United States to other countries find the United States lacks healthcare quality, particularly on issues related to equity and access.[2,3] Using the car example above, the United States is getting "lemon" quality while paying a luxury car price. The concept of *value*, generally defined as *quality* divided by *cost*, is used to describe this fundamental problem of the U.S.

healthcare system. Current healthcare reform efforts, such as *value-based purchasing* and *ACOs*, focus on efforts to maximize value by improving quality while simultaneously reducing costs. These efforts impact both community pharmacists and hospital pharmacists directly through *performance-based payment* models. Regardless of setting, quality has become a feature of pharmacy practice today.

## ■ COMMON KEY CONCEPTS IN HEALTHCARE QUALITY

When thinking about healthcare quality measures, it is helpful to think about it in terms of a framework. Donabedian's structure, process, and outcome (SPO) model is a common categorization scheme (Table 10-1).[4] *Structure* pertains to tangible or intangible static attributes of the healthcare system. How this structure is used to provide care pertains to *process*. *Outcome* relates to the ultimate goals of care provided. For example, let's think about a patient coming to the community pharmacy setting and meeting with a pharmacist who has obtained the Certified Diabetes Educator (CDE) credential. The CDE credential and patient's blood glucose meter are both structural elements of healthcare. The patient's use of their medication and the pharmacist's skill in caring for the patient are both processes. Since we are thinking about this scenario in terms of diabetes, ultimate patient care goals would be focused on overall wellness and avoiding macro- and microvascular complications. Specific markers used to monitor disease progression, such as hemoglobin A1c, are considered outcomes, as are events which patients would like to avoid such as hospitalizations. Patient perceptions of quality include satisfaction with the care they have received.

All quality measures include a denominator and a numerator. The denominator is the patient population we want to measure. It is developed using inclusion and exclusion criteria for a specific patient population. For example, let's use adherence to non-insulin diabetes medications. The patient population we are focusing on are patients who have type 2 diabetes that are at least 18 years old, enrolled in a health plan, and have filled

**Table 10-1. Key Quality Concepts**

| Concept | Description |
|---|---|
| Structural measure | Quality measure assessing a physical attribute of a healthcare system that supports care quality. Examples include pharmacist credentials, hours the pharmacy is open, and specific capacities of a pharmacy management system. |
| Process measure | Quality measure assessing the use of a healthcare structure to provide quality care. Examples include prescribing of guideline-recommended therapy, comprehensive medication review completion rates, and percentage of patients adherence to a medication. |
| Outcome measure | Quality measure assessing ultimate goals of care. Includes patient-reported outcomes and satisfaction, as well as major events like disease progression, avoidable hospitalizations, and mortality. Examples include percent of patients with an hemoglobin A1c (HbA1c) >9% and percent of patients admitted to the hospital for an avoidable diabetes-related complication. |
| Denominator | Population targeted for a given quality measure. |
| Numerator | The quality concept evaluated for the target population. For measures like comprehensive medication review completion rate and adherence where a positive score is better, patients who fail to meet numerator criteria count against a pharmacy's performance score. These patients are often referred to as outliers. |
| Attribution | The process of assigning patients to pharmacies and other entities for the purposes of identifying who is responsible for the patient's care. A patient could be attributed to different pharmacies depending on the specific measure being assessed. |
| Proportion of days covered (PDC) | Used to measure medication adherence calculated by dividing the number of days in period "covered" by a medication based on dispensed quantity divided by the number of days in the period. A patient is considered adherent if they have >0.8 or 80% of days covered by a medication during a defined period. |

2 or more non-insulin diabetes medications, i.e., inclusion criteria. Patients who are on insulin would be excluded from this measure, i.e., exclusion criteria. The numerator looks at what we want to measure. In the case of this example, the numerator includes patients who have at least 80% of days during the specific measurement period covered by non-insulin diabetes medications. A specific term for this method of calculating adherence is *proportion of days covered* (PDC). To calculate the PDC, the total number of days covered by prescription refills in a given measurement period is divided by the number of days between the first fill and the end of the measurement period. As an example, "J.D." fills a prescription of 30 tablets 11 times between January 1 and December 31. The first fill was January

9. This spans 330 days covered by refills out of a total of 356 days from the period January 9 to December 31. This results in 93% of days covered.[5]

To calculate a performance score for an individual pharmacy or other entity, each specific patient score is aggregated. However, before this can be done, patients first need to be attributed to the pharmacy or other entity who will be responsible for their care. There are 2 different ways a patient can be attributed to a pharmacy—through an encounter or an event. An example of an encounter would be a patient visiting the pharmacy and picking up medications. In this type of *attribution*, the patient would be attributed to the pharmacy that provides the most care to the patient in a given timeframe. You might be thinking, "what happens if a patient lives in New York and spends the winters in Florida?" If the patient has more encounters at the pharmacy in New York than the pharmacy in Florida in a given timeframe, the patient would be attributed to the Florida pharmacy. It is important to note that this is all dependent on the timeframe that the measure is looking at. The second type of attribution is through an event. In this case, a certain trigger happens such as an emergency medical situation. The pharmacy who handles the situation would get the credit and the patient would be attributed to them.[6]

## ■ USE OF QUALITY MEASURES WITHIN PERFORMANCE-BASED PAYMENT MODELS

Performance-based payment model design widely varies. Two major types of models are accountable care organizations (ACOs) and pay-for-performance models. ACOs encourage coordination between outpatient and inpatient service providers to incentivize reductions in healthcare spending and share savings with groups who meet specific quality benchmarks. Pay-for-performance models use quality and spending measures to evaluate performance and determine bonuses or penalties linked to performance. Community pharmacists can influence quality and cost within each model.

## ■ PERFORMANCE-BASED PAYMENT MODELS FOR COMMUNITY PHARMACISTS

More than 42 million patients are in a performance-based program managed by pharmacists.[7] Performance-based payments make up a larger percentage of community pharmacies' revenue when compared to previous years. With decreasing margins on prescriptions, community pharmacies—especially independent pharmacies—who do not perform well in these models could experience financial difficulties. To make things even more complicated, each model varies between payers. This can cause challenges for community pharmacists as they are required to manage performance for each plan, which might have a different set of measures.

Medicare has 4 parts: Part A, Part B, Part C, and Part D. Part A provides patients inpatient or hospital coverage. Part B is outpatient coverage which include screenings, primary care, and some procedures. Part C, also known as Medicare Advantage Plans, are how some patients choose to get their benefits through private insurers. Lastly, Part D is an optional prescription drug benefit that patients can enroll in. In 2008, Centers for Medicare and Medicaid Services (CMS) implemented the Medicare Stars Rating program to measure quality of care.[8] This program relies on quality measures to evaluate performance at the plan-level for Medicare Part C and Part D plans. A 5-star system is used to rate plans, and Part C plans can receive bonus payments if they achieve a score of 4 or more stars. For each plan, measures related to medications make up 40% of the Part D Stars Rating score. It is important to note that while plans receive a rating based on the 5-star system, pharmacies do not receive a rating from Medicare. Measures commonly used in performance-based payment models for Medicare are: adherence to renin-angiotensin system antagonists (RASA), adherence to statins, adherence to non-insulin diabetes medications, statin use in diabetes, and comprehensive medication review completion rates (Table 10-2).[9]

Plans can incentivize community pharmacy performance in one of 3 ways: rewards, penalties, or a mix of both rewards and penalties. In the *rewards-based model*, community pharmacies which exceed certain benchmarks on included performance measures receive bonus payments. One challenge with this type of model is having a large enough bonus for pharmacies to pursue. For example, a community pharmacy can make an additional $20 000 in bonuses by meeting certain adherence-related performance goals. However, to meet these goals, they would have to invest ≥$20 000 in additional staff or new technology. A pharmacy manager or owner might not find that the cost justifies the reward. While a health plan might view $20 000 as a large bonus, it might not be large enough for the community pharmacist to respond to the incentive.[10]

**Table 10-2. Common Quality Measures Used in Performance-Based Payment Model for Medicare**

| Description | Denominator | Numerator |
| --- | --- | --- |
| Adherence to renin-angiotensin system antagonists (RASA) | Patients aged 65 years or older with at least 2 fills of RASA medications during the measurement year. | Patients in the denominator with PDC greater than or equal to 80%. |
| Adherence to statins | Patients aged 65 or older with at least 2 fills of statin medications during the measurement year. | Patients in the denominator with PDC greater than or equal to 80%. |
| Adherence to non-insulin diabetes medications | Patients aged 65 or older with at least 2 fills of non-insulin diabetes medications across any eligible class during the measurement year. Patients filling insulin are excluded. | Patients in the denominator with PDC greater than or equal to 80%. |
| Statin use in persons with diabetes | Patients aged 40–75 dispensed at least 2 diabetes medications. | Patients in the denominator who filled at least one statin medication. |
| Comprehensive medication review completion rate | Patients aged 18 and older who are enrolled in a Medication Therapy Management Program. | Patients in the denominator who received a comprehensive medication review. |

Many plans, especially Medicare Part D plans, use the *penalty-based model* when implementing performance-based payment models. As compared to the rewards-based model, this model does not reward those who meet specific goals. Instead, it penalizes those who do not meet those specific goals. In Medicare, these penalties are applied through direct and indirect remuneration (DIR) fees.[11] DIR fees are not new, but the use of this mechanism in performance-based payments has increased substantially in recent years. Medicare plan sponsors use DIR fees to recoup payments made to community pharmacies for prescription drugs.

As previously mentioned, some plans use a mix of both rewards for high performers and penalties for low performers; however this is very rare. For almost all Medicare plans, community pharmacies with high performance have lower DIR fees than community pharmacies with lower performance. However, both pharmacies still have to pay DIR fees due to fixed fees tied with participation in a network. These fees often leave pharmacies with little explanation for the large bill. This has caused frustration among community pharmacists—specifically pharmacy owners—as they feel these fees are unavoidable.

## ■ STRATEGIES TO IMPROVE PERFORMANCE SCORES

While performance-based payment models might seem overwhelming at first, there are several strategies that can be implemented to improve performance (Table 10-3) that will ultimately lead to reduced DIR fees and improved patient outcomes. The first step to improving quality measures is to pay attention. You should know your pharmacy scores and which measures are included in third party contracts. Almost

| Table 10-3. | Strategies to Improve Performance Scores |
|---|---|
| **Strategy** | **Description** |
| Monitor quality scores | Use the EQuIPP platform or another vendor to monitor quality scores regularly. The most engaged pharmacies often check their scores weekly or even more frequently. Additionally, for pharmacies which are a part of a regional or national chain, these quality scores may be included in key performance indicators and monitored at the corporate level. |
| Identify a quality champion | Designate a specific individual to take charge of quality initiatives and monitor quality. This could be a pharmacist, pharmacy technician, student pharmacist, or other pharmacy staff members. |
| Create a culture of continuous quality improvement | Culture is key. To maximize performance, a culture of quality improvement is needed to align all staff members to the idea that ongoing change is needed to improve quality. Success is less likely if quality improvement is left up to the quality champion alone. |
| Implement specific services | Identify areas of weakness and implement specific services to address it. For example, many interventions exist to improve adherence rates, such as medication synchronization and 90-day medication fills. |
| Target outliers | EQuIPP and other vendors provide outlier reports which can identify patients who are negatively affecting quality scores. Target outreach to these patients. If the number of outliers is large, consider targeting patients closest to meeting quality score (e.g., target an outlier with 75% adherence vs 50% adherence). |
| Collaborate with other healthcare providers | Measures used for pharmacists are starting to be used to measure care quality for physicians and other healthcare providers. Additionally, measures typically used to evaluate physicians, such as A1c control, are starting to be used to evaluate pharmacy performance. This increasing crossover of quality measures should increase the willingness for other providers to collaborate with pharmacists on shared quality goals. |

all Part D plan sponsors use a platform developed by Pharmacy Quality Solutions to calculate performance for performance-based payment models.[7] This platform is called the Electronic Quality Improvement Platform for Plans and Pharmacies (EQuIPP™). It has a portal for pharmacies to log into which displays measure scores for specific plans as well as identifies patients who might be outliers for a specific measure.

Keep in mind that performance information is reconciled over time on the EQuIPP platform, which means claims that are reversed or resubmitted will be reflected in the performance score. Proper billing is of the utmost importance—whenever a pharmacy bills a claim to another carrier, discount card, or fills for cash,

those claims do not make it to the insurance carrier, and the pharmacy does not receive credit. As a result, performance scores can be negatively impacted.

Strategies to improve patient-level performance depend on the measure—there is not one specific strategy that will fit all measures. Also what works for one community pharmacy might not work for another. It is important for pharmacy staff, pharmacists, and pharmacy technicians, to assess their workflow to identify areas for improvement and strategies to address identified gaps.

One strategy commonly used to improve medication adherence is medication synchronization.[12] When implementing medication synchronization, medication fills are aligned to the same day of the month. A pick up time is scheduled for all medications. Some medication synchronization programs also align medication pick up with a clinically-oriented appointment where medication-related therapy problems are addressed. The latter is referred to the appointment-based model which is a best practice.[13,14,15] While some studies show improvement in medication adherence when implementing medication synchronization, the results are not consistent across studies. Some community pharmacies have combined their medication synchronization program with medication packaging such as bubble or blister packs and this strategy has improved medication adherence.[16]

Another strategy to improve performance scores is implementing 90-day medication fills. While changing from 30-day to 90-day fills can increase the PDC and in turn improve adherence scores, it is uncertain if this actually creates better adherence or improved outcomes.[17] When considering switching to 90-day medication fills, it is important to take into consideration: (1) individual needs of your patient and (2) cost of the medication. Patients who might benefit from 90-day medication fills are those who have transportation issues or rely on a caregiver to pick up medications. Patients who might benefit from 30-day medication fills include those with lower health literacy to provide frequent medication education or those who warrant motivation to stay on track. The monthly touch-points with pharmacy staff could be beneficial to helping improve their adherence. The cost of the medication should also be considered when determining if you are going to fill a 90-day supply. Some patients' insurance plan might charge the same copay for a 30-day supply as they would for a 90-day supply. If a patient is struggling with affording their medication, this might be a good option.

Another way to improve adherence to medications is through home delivery. For patients who are home-bound or those who have difficulty obtaining transportation, this can be very impactful. While home delivery programs are common among independent pharmacies, large chain pharmacies have started partnering with delivery companies to provide this service to their patients.[18]

When thinking about measures that are not related to medication adherence such as statin use in persons with diabetes, it is important to make sure strong relationships exist between the community pharmacist and prescriber. For a patient with diabetes to start a new prescription for a statin, the pharmacist would have to contact a prescriber for initiation of a new prescription. Having strong relationships with local prescribers can have an impact on whether the recommendation for a new statin is accepted or not.[19]

Lastly when thinking about strategies to improve performance scores, it is important to make sure you are checking patient outliers on EQuIPP™. By looking at each outlier's PDC, you can identify which patients to target to improve adherence. For example, you realize that you only need 2 more patients to achieve a PDC threshold of 80% or higher to meet a goal set by a plan. You should first target 2 patients whose PDC is closest to meeting 80%. Then, target the rest of the outliers. While we want to make sure we are reaching out to all of our nonadherent patients, prioritization of outliers is also an important strategy.

For additional information on increasing pharmacy value through the incorporation of clinical services as well as how to implement Medication Therapy Management services, see Chapter 11, "Clinical and Value-Based Services."

## ■ SUMMARY

Now let's think back to the example we provided at the beginning of the chapter about taking your car to the mechanic. Throughout this chapter, we discussed the changes in the United States' healthcare system from a fee-for-service model to a value-based model. If we were to relate the car mechanic example to taking care of patients, the value-based model would be very similar to having a warranty on a part or specific service. Community pharmacies are now being held accountable for not only the prescriptions they fill but also a patient's outcomes and quality of care received regardless of how much they were initially paid for a prescription or service. By focusing on ways to improve performance scores, community pharmacists can maximize both patient care and revenue.

# ■ CHAPTER APPLICATIONS

1. Imagine you are a community pharmacist who wants to improve their care for patients with diabetes. How could you change structural elements to improve healthcare quality?

2. Look up the current list of quality measures included in the Medicare Star Ratings program for Medicare Part D. Which of the measures can the pharmacist have the greatest impact on? Least impact on? How do these measures compare to the list of measures in Table 10-2?

3. Imagine you are on a rotation of Advanced Pharmacy Practice Experience with Patients First Pharmacy. Your project for the month is putting together a plan for how to improve their EQuIPP scores. Using Table 10-3, what should be included in your plan to improve Patients First Pharmacy's performance scores?

4. Your approach for the project includes identifying patients with diabetes who have statin adherence between 70% and 79% and calling them to see if they need refills. How would you implement this process?

5. After identifying and reaching out to the non-adherent patients, you realize a lot of patients don't have a car and only get their medication filled when a friend can pick them up and bring them to them. What are some solutions for these patients to improve their adherence?

# REFERENCES

1. Centers for Medicare and Medicaid Services. National Health Expenditure Fact Sheet. Published 2020. Updated March 24. Accessed May 11, 2020. https://www.cms.gov/Research-Statistics-Data-and-Systems/Statistics-Trends-and-Reports/National HealthExpendData/NHE-Fact-Sheet

2. Schneider E, Sarnak D, Squires D, Shah A, Doty M. Mirror, Mirror 2017: International Comparison Reflects Flaws and Opportunities for Better US Health Care. The Commonwealth Fund; July 2017. Accessed December 13, 2021. https://australiangpalliance.com.au/wp-content/uploads/2018/05/Schneider_mirror_mirror_2017.pdf

3. Organisation for Economic Cooperation and Development (OECD). Health at a Glance 2019: OECD Indicators. OECD; November 7, 2019. Accessed December 13, 2021. doi.org/10.1787/4dd50c09-en

4. Donabedian A. The quality of care. How can it be assessed? *JAMA*. 1988;260(12):1743–1748.

5. Schwartz L, Reese D, Rogers A. Quality Measures. America's Pharmacist. Alexandria, VA: National Community Pharmacists Association; June 2014.

6. Pharmacy Quality Solutions. Understanding Quality Measure Calculations in Your EQuIPP Dashboard. November 15, 2016. Accessed May 26, 2021. https://www.pharmacyquality.com/wp-content/uploads/2018/08/EQuIPPMeasureCalc.pdf

7. Pharmacy Quality Solutions. Pharmacy Quality Solutions Web Site. Published 2021. Accessed January 28, 2021. https://www.pharmacyquality.com/

8. Centers for Medicare and Medicaid Services. Fact Sheet – 2020 Part C and D Star Ratings. October 10, 2019. Accessed May 26, 2021. https://www.cms.gov/Medicare/Prescription-Drug-Coverage/PrescriptionDrugCovGenIn/Downloads/2020-Star-Ratings-Fact-Sheet-.pdf

9. Pharmacy Quality Alliance. Medicare 2020 Star Ratings Update. November 7, 2019. https://vimeo.com/372977183

10. Urick B RC, Pathak S, Livet M, Jackson J. Structure and implementation environment of performance-based pharmacy payment models. *J Manag Care Pharm*. 2020;26(10-a).

11. National Community Pharmacists Association. Frequently Asked Questions (FAQs) About Pharmacy "DIR" Fees. National Community Pharmacists Association; August 5, 2019. http://www.ncpa.co/pdf/dir-faq.pdf

12. Patti M, Renfro CP, Posey R, Wu G, Turner K, Ferreri SP. Systematic review of medication synchronization in community pharmacy practice. *Res Social Adm Pharm*. 2019;15(11):1281–1288.

13. Holdford D, Saxena K. Impact of appointment-based medication synchronization on existing users of chronic medications. *J Manag Care Spec Pharm*. 2015;21(8):662–669.

14. Holdford DA, Inocencio TJ. Adherence and persistence associated with an appointment-based medication synchronization program. *J Am Pharm Assoc (2003)*. 2013;53(6):576–583.

15. Dao N, Lee S, Hata M, Sarino L. Impact of appointment-based medication synchronization on proportion of days covered for chronic medications. *Pharmacy (Basel)*. 2018;6(2):44.

16. Aarons GA, Green AE, Palinkas LA, et al. Dynamic adaptation process to implement an evidence-based child maltreatment intervention. *Implement Sci*. 2012;7(32):32.

17. Farley J, Urick BY, Schondelmeyer S. Letter—Community pharmacy versus mail order: An uneven comparison. *J Manag Care Spec Pharm*. 2019 Jun;25(6):724-725.

18. CVS Pharmacy Launches Same-Day, On-Demand Rx Delivery Nationwide. Press Release. April 4, 2019. Accessed May 26, 2021. https://cvshealth.com/newsroom/press-releases/cvs-pharmacy-launches-same-day-demand-rx-delivery-nationwide

19. Renner HM, Hollar A, Stolpe SF, Marciniak MW. Pharmacist-to-prescriber intervention to close therapeutic gaps for statin use in patients with diabetes: A randomized controlled trial. *J Am Pharm Assoc (2003)*. 2017;57(3, Supplement):S236–S242.e231.

# 11

# CLINICAL AND VALUE-BASED SERVICES

*Angelina Tucker, PharmD, BCGP, and Roxane L. Took, PharmD, BCACP*

---

## ▧ LEARNING OBJECTIVES

1. Describe the misalignment of community pharmacy value expression and the concept of clinical integration.
2. Compare and contrast current and emerging models for clinical services and their payment in the community pharmacy setting.
3. Create a new clinical service implementation plan using community pharmacy practice transformation domains from the Flip the Pharmacy program.

The healthcare environment is changing dramatically. Pharmacy chains are expanding and non-pharmacy entities are entering the pharmacy space (e.g., Amazon purchasing Pillpack©). Reimbursement for medications have drastically decreased over the last decade. Alternative payment models for enhanced services at the pharmacy, separate from the product, are essential to the financial well-being of the pharmacy. Enhanced services increase the quality of care provided to patients and positively impact quality metrics for both physicians and insurance plans.

You are the pharmacy manager of an independent pharmacy located in a small town. Large chain pharmacies are moving in and trying to buy your pharmacy and others in the area. Your pharmacy owner wants to sell the pharmacy due to increasing direct and indirect remuneration (DIR) fees. This change has forced the pharmacy to sell many medications below cost. In the past 6 months, many patients have transferred to competitors because your pharmacy was not in their insurance's preferred network. Because you are no longer in-network, their prescriptions were no longer covered at your pharmacy. You have recently graduated from pharmacy school and convinced the owner to offer value-based services as an alternative payment model to help the pharmacy stay local and in business.

## ■ MISALIGNMENT OF VALUE EXPRESSION

In the past 5 years, several news headlines have reflected the drastic changes in the healthcare environment due to a reduction in reimbursements for the dispensing of medications. Rite Aid sold 2186 pharmacies to Walgreens in 2017,[1] Walgreens laid off an undisclosed number of employees in an effort to save more than $1.8 billion in expenses in 2019,[2] and CVS announced plans to close 22 stores in 2020. If large chain pharmacies are downsizing, this leaves little hope for smaller, independent pharmacy owners. Access, quality, and cost make up the components of current payment models. Improving 1 or 2 components will inevitably result in the expense of the third. It becomes evident that the fast, accurate, affordable business model of the big pharmacy chains is not sustainable, hence the urgency for payment reform in the community pharmacy setting.

Of the entire U.S. healthcare budget, pharmacy contributes 10% of spending while medical costs (e.g., emergency department [ED] visits, hospitalizations, diagnostics, and ambulance services) account for 90%.[3] Pharmacists can impact these medical costs by identifying and resolving medication-related problems while providing disease state education. Thus, there arises a misalignment in the value expression of pharmacists in the current payment model. These services keep the patients healthy and out of the hospital, hence decreasing healthcare spending. Pharmacy services impact the medical costs, yet pharmacy payment only comes from the 10% set aside for pharmacy and outpatient medicine dispensing.

Value expression at the community pharmacies is currently based on dispensing medications. However, the demand for improved health outcomes and meeting quality metrics is the impetus for new value-based payment models in pharmacy. The current model of "quick, accurate and affordable" medication dispensing is not a sustainable business model. Do note, that fee-for-service (FFS) tasks like dispensing medications can have incredible value if coupled with pay-for-performance (P4P) services in a patient care model with disease management.

### Clinically Integrated Network (CIN) of Pharmacies

A CIN consists of a group of healthcare providers that work together to facilitate the coordination of patient care across conditions, providers, and settings to improve patient care and decrease overall healthcare costs.[4] Clinical integration allows community pharmacies to join a larger network that can collectively negotiate to sell services to payers including healthcare plans, employers, and government sponsors.[5]

In the pharmacy setting, the Community Pharmacy Enhanced Services Network (CPESN) is the only available CIN. Pharmacies, as part of CPESN, can work directly with payers (e.g., healthcare plans, accountable care organizations [ACOs]) to engage in value-based contracting. CPESN can consist of a CIN of competing pharmacy providers (i.e., combination of independent pharmacies, regional chains, national chains) or exist as a completely financially integrated national chain pharmacy organization, both of which are viewed equally in function to a prospective payer and capable of providing high quality care while accepting financial risks. CPESN collects data from these pharmacies across the United States to show how pharmacies can improve quality outcomes. By collecting data, CPESN can create a pharmacy equivalent of an ACO.

For example, CPESN can contract with a medical plan in a P4P model to receive bonus payment if the pharmacies within CPESN reduce targeted patients A1c to less than 9%. In this model, the pharmacies will also be financially penalized (or accepting risk) if they are unable to decrease to the targeted A1c. Collectively pharmacies within CPESN can negotiate with plans and payers who recognize the value of the pharmacist's ability to lower costs associated with reduced blood glucose, decreased hospitalizations, improved employee productivity, decreased ER visits, and other medical-related problems. Pharmacies also have the option of contracting with plans individually in a P4P model.

## Pharmacy Quality Alliance (PQA)

PQA was established in 2006. It is a nongovernmental organization partnering with the Centers for Medicare and Medicaid Services (CMS) to develop quality measures. These measures are routinely updated but currently include the four categories of adherence, appropriate medication use, medication safety and medication management services. For an updated list of the specific measures within these categories visit the Pharmacy Quality Alliance website. The Electronic Quality Improvement Platform for Plans and Pharmacies (EQuIPP®) is the platform used by PQA to manage the performance data available to both health plans and pharmacy organizations.

The quality measures for "adherence" are typically measured by calculating the *proportion of days covered (PDC)* based on quantity of medications dispensed and timing of prescription refill. The PDC threshold is the level above which the medication has a reasonable likelihood of achieving the most clinical benefit. Clinical evidence provides support for a standard PDC threshold of 80%;[6] however, pharmacies may have more stringent adherence goals. The "appropriate medication use" quality metric is related to indication and effectiveness, e.g., needing a statin therapy in patients diagnosed with diabetes. The "medication safety" quality metric is related to high-risk medications, e.g., anticholinergic use in patients >65 years of age. Annual *comprehensive medication review (CMR)* completion rate is another quality metric used. For more detail, refer to Chapter 10, "Quality Metrics."

## Electronic Quality Improvement Platform for Plans and Pharmacies (EQuIPP®)

EQuIPP® is an online platform used to help community pharmacies identify their performance. The platform has a performance dashboard that rates pharmacies based on each of the PQA quality measures.[7] For example, EQuIPP® may identify a pharmacy's goal as concurrent use of opioids and benzodiazepines should be less than 10% for all patients at the pharmacy. If the pharmacy is not at goal, the platform will identify patients (aka outliers) that are concurrently using both opioids and benzodiazepines. Pharmacists can take action based on the information provided in EQuIPP® to reach their goal. Pharmacies meeting and exceeding these goals will earn a 5-star rating. Pharmacies performing at the top 20% are able to be a part of a preferred pharmacy network with insurance plans. See Chapter 10, "Quality Metrics" for in-depth description and strategies on improving performance scores.

# THE CURRENT MODEL FOR CLINICAL SERVICES AND REIMBURSEMENT

## Reimbursement Models

Below are various reimbursement models that are available in the community pharmacy setting for value-based clinical services. For additional information, see Chapter 9, "Payment Models and Methods."

1. *FFS*: This payment model is based on payment for a specific service, e.g., A1c test or colonoscopy. This type of payment model is rapidly falling out of favor not only due to ACA and MACRA but also due to the fact that it does not align pharmacy incentives with the provider's performance. This model pays for the intervention not the outcome, e.g., completion of an A1c test every 6 months versus the goal quality measure of A1c < 9%. Payment can be made separate from the product, e.g., medication therapy management (MTM) billing, or it can be paid as part of the product, e.g., service fee for administration of a long-acting antipsychotic.

2. *Per-member-per-month (PMPM) or per-member-per-year (PMPY)*: Insurers using this capitated payment model provide a fixed amount of funds per member per period of time to the pharmacy up front. The pharmacy, instead of the insurer, uses these funds to cover the costs of the patient's medications and pharmacy-related services. This model can be beneficial for patients that underutilize medications and services; however, it can result in a net loss to the pharmacy if patients require excessive medications and services.

   Per member can be interpreted differently depending on:
   - Targeted member: for example, high-risk chronic heart failure (CHF) patient, e.g., $10.00 per member
   - Enrolled Member: for example, there are 1000 members in the plan but 100 have CHF
   - Employed Member: number of employees versus dependents
   - Dependent Members

3. *P4P*: Remuneration is subject to outcome metrics. For example, it can be based on:
   - Process: for example, colonoscopies outcomes
   - Clinical: for example, A1c < 9%, BP < 140/90 mmHg
   - Global: 30-day hospital readmission rates
   - Humanistic- Patient reported outcomes: for example, Consumer Assessment of Healthcare Providers and Systems (CAHPS)

   For additional information, see Chapter 10, "Quality Metrics."

4. *Hybrid*: This model refers to many different methods of payments used to create alignment between pharmacy providers, payers, purchasers, and partners. The method holds the pharmacy accountable for achieving a specific measure by putting their reimbursements at risk.
   - Combination of FFS and P4P
     - For example, the pharmacy is paid for an A1c test every 4 months but will incur additional bonus payments if it is <9%.
   - Withhold: The pharmacy is paid a fee for service, but if an outcome is met, the pharmacy can obtain the full payment from the insurance/payer.
     - For example, the pharmacy is paid $50 per patient for blood pressure (BP) monitoring, but $10 of that payment would be withheld until the performance measure of BP < 130/80 mmHg is met.
   - Different FFS rates based on performance
     - For example, $10 for a patient achieving a weight loss < 5%, $15 for weight loss < 7%, $20 for weight loss < 10%.
   - Bonus payments based on performance: Initial payments are based upon the capitated model, but pharmacies can also obtain bonus payments if they meet and exceed predetermined metrics (e.g., achieving a weight loss goal of 7% over 6 months or smoking cessation).
   - Shared savings: If the pharmacy meets predetermined metrics and the plan receives bonuses based on these metrics, both the pharmacy and the plan will share this bonus.

- PMPM and P4P: Different payment rates based on performance
  - For example, for a pharmacy at a gold level they will receive $2.54 if they are able to meet metrics; if a pharmacy is at the silver level, they will receive $2.10; at the bronze level, the pharmacy will receive $1.50; and for pharmacies below bronze level they will not receive payment.
  - Bonus FFS based on performance
    - For example, pharmacies can receive a PMPM for engaging a patient in diabetes counselling but 80% bonus if the patients meet the target A1C < 9%.
  - Shared savings baseline: If the payer meets their baseline quality metric and receive bonus payments at the end of the year, then they will share a percentage of these savings with the pharmacy.

## Pharmacist-Administered Immunizations

As trusted and highly accessible healthcare providers, pharmacists are well positioned to increase the public's access to immunizations. The first organized immunization training for a group of 50 pharmacists was held in Seattle, Washington, in late 1994. By 1995, 9 states allowed pharmacists to immunize, and in 1996, the American Pharmacists Association (APhA) began its nationally recognized immunization training program for pharmacists.[8] Currently, all 50 states allow pharmacists to administer vaccinations, with Maine being the last state to allow pharmacists to administer immunizations in 2009.[9] Specific details regarding the pharmacist's authority to administer vaccines is determined by each state's laws and regulations.

Flu clinics are an excellent form of community marketing and engagement. A pharmacist can position themselves to not only promote goodwill and a valuable service to the community, but also advertise their pharmacy to increase customer retention and acquisition. A potential partnership with third party payors is particularly advantageous to help decrease sick days and decrease health plan costs by helping reduce the incidence of flu in members who receive a flu vaccine.

## Pharmacy-Based Travel Health Services

In 2019, there were approximately 45,000 international travelers from the United States, representing a 7% increase from the previous year.[10] A questionnaire administered at the John F. Kennedy International Airport found that although many travelers believed that vaccination was effective for prevention, yet very few indicated they were vaccinated before their travels.[11] This represents a growing need to expand access and increase awareness of travel health vaccination. Pharmacists can play a vital role in disease prevention and education related to international travel and health risks. Travel health services vary from state to state based on the scope of practice and legislation, but can include screening, counseling, administering vaccines, obtaining prescription medications, ordering/interpreting laboratory tests, and providing self-care medications.[12] Immunizations can be billed at the pharmacy as a FFS through Medicare Parts B and D coverage.

## Medication Therapy Management (MTM)

MTM is a patient-centered, comprehensive approach to improve medication use, reduce the risk of adverse events, and improve medication adherence.[13] Therefore, the programs include high-touch interventions to engage the beneficiary and their prescribers. Some electronic platforms used to document these interventions include OutcomesMTM®, RxCompanion™, and OptumRx® MedMonitor.

OutcomesMTM® is the most common electronic platform used by community pharmacists to identify patients eligible for MTM services and stratify them according to health risks. MTM can be extensive, as in a CMR, or more selective for a specific disease state or medication, as in a *targeted intervention program (TIP)*.[13] A CMR is a patient interview process with the pharmacist, utilizing the patient care process to optimize health and medication outcomes.[14] Using the principles of evidence-based practice, pharmacists collect, assess, plan, implement, and follow-up in collaboration with the patient's other healthcare providers. When conducting a CMR, pharmacists schedule an appointment with the patient to update health conditions, identify medication-related problems, create an updated medication list, and build an action plan for any problems identified.

Medicare Part D Plan sponsors are required to offer MTM services to patients who meet specified criteria. In 2021 Medicare patients are eligible for MTM services if they meet the following criteria: 3 or more specified multiple chronic conditions, multiple medications, and an estimated annual drug cost of $4376 or more.[15] This information is updated annually and may be found at the CMS webpage on MTM.[15] By completing specified targeted interventions and CMRs, pharmacies can earn higher performance scores.[16] Performance scores indicate how your pharmacy compares to all other MTM centers.

A pharmacist unsure of how to begin delivering clinical services can start with a TIP. TIPs focus on medication safety, adherence, and appropriate use of medications. For example, the pharmacies will receive an alert from the MTM platform to target patients with diabetes who are 40–75 years old without a prescribed statin on file. Pharmacists will be prompted to contact the patient's prescriber for initiation of statin therapy. A workflow process to incorporate MTM services at the pharmacy can follow the implementation process outlined in the "Step-by-Step Community Pharmacy Practice Transformation" section later in this chapter.

PDC as a star measure can be increased through converting patients from 30-day to 90-day fills, synchronizing a patient's chronic medications to be filled on the same day (aka medication synchronization or med sync) or using compliance packaging.[17–19] Through MTM, pharmacies can increase PDC scores, generate revenue for the pharmacy through billing via MTM platforms, and potentially, lower DIR fees by increasing the pharmacy's Medicare star rating which can result in additional reimbursements based on their performance.

## ◼ THE EVOLUTION OF CLINICAL SERVICES IN THE COMMUNITY PHARMACY

Pharmacists can demonstrate their value to the public and the healthcare system by initiating clinical programs within the community pharmacy setting. In order to meet the needs of the community, it is important to identify both the health and the social issues most prevalent in that community. This could include conversations with local health authorities and medical providers or reviewing community needs' assessment surveys. Additionally, it may be helpful to conduct an analysis of the population at the county level using resources such as the U.S. census report (census.gov), National Center for Health Statistics (cdc.gov/nchs), and county-specific websites (e.g., countyhealthrankings.org), which can be used to find demographics, prevalence of certain health conditions, social determinants of health, etc. Other useful data include the number and type of prescriptions filled to evaluate local prescribing patterns as well as health outcomes measures from local physician groups and hospitals. After reviewing local data, clinical services and programs can be created based on the needs of the population. By meeting the needs of both the patients and the medical providers of the local community, pharmacies can demonstrate their value to patients and healthcare providers through reducing healthcare costs and improving health outcomes.

For example, a pharmacy in a local community with a large percentage of the "super sick" category can develop their clinical service by collaborating with local hospitals and physicians. The "super sick" population typically consists of those with 5 or more chronic conditions; hence, the disease management services may include diabetes self-management education, *transitions of care (TOC)*, or behavioral health programs. Specialized clinical services can effectively target this population to not only increase quality care but also result in a financially sustainable service through medical billing. However, a pharmacy located in a college town will undoubtedly have a different demographic with different needs than the community in the previous example. Such a town may have a population that is largely healthy with no chronic conditions, so services that benefit this population would focus on disease prevention rather than disease management. Services offered in this community could include immunization clinics, travel vaccine clinics, smoking cessation, weight loss programs, sexually transmitted disease testing and education, and depression screening.

The increased need for clinical services also resulted in a need for an improved format for documenting these encounters and interventions. The eCare plan is a standardized method for documenting patient encounters.[20] This allows pharmacists to document in the same format as physicians in order to retrieve and collate data for value-based payments, which are payments for enhanced clinical services. The eCare plans address the longitudinal care of the patient over a period of time as various factors affect the current disease state which is the basis of P4P. This differs from the current claims data which captures information about the patient at one moment in time or a FFS model.[20] A template for an eCare plan can be found at https://www.ecareplaninitiative.com/

## Pharmacist-Provided Collaborative Care Services

Pharmacists may develop contracts or *collaborative practice agreements (CPA)* with physicians to provide various collaborative care services. The CPA is a formal agreement in which a licensed provider makes a diagnosis, supervises patient care, and refers patients to a pharmacist under a protocol that allows the pharmacist to perform specific patient care functions. Each state has explicit laws governing this agreement.

Pharmacists are typically reimbursed through prescription insurance for medications or MTM services. Pharmacies can also bill medical insurance for other limited services that include immunizations and durable medical equipment. That said, pharmacists may need to contract with physicians to provide various collaborative care services based on state laws. Although pharmacists can be used to provide this

service, the medical billing must ultimately be completed by a physician.

Physicians may delegate healthcare professionals to perform services to Medicare patients under their supervision and provide a mechanism for billing such services, which is referred to as *incident-to-billing*.[21,22] Although pharmacists may provide certain services, incident-to-billing must be submitted to medical plans by a physician. There are other billing methods available, and it is dependent upon services provided, location of services delivered, and pharmacists' scope of practice as determined by the state board of pharmacy.

Physicians may negotiate specific contracts with private payers that outline a method for payment to provide reimbursement for patient care services provided by pharmacists. Alternatively, pharmacist services may be included in payment models or associated with P4P incentives. Examples include value-based care models via the Quality Payment Program that rewards the delivery of high-quality patient care through the Merit-Based Incentive Payment System (MIPS) and advanced alternative payment models.[23]

There are many preventive and screening services that are covered by Medicare Part B that may be offered to beneficiaries by a pharmacist in collaboration with a physician or group. These include cardiovascular disease screening and behavioral therapy, depression screening, diabetes screening and self-management training, immunizations, nutrition therapy services, hepatitis B and C screening, HIV screening, obesity screening and counseling, screening and counselling for sexually transmitted diseases/infections, tobacco use cessation counseling, and annual wellness visits.[24-26] Pharmacists may form contractual agreements with physician offices to provide the above services, and billing may be done via incident-to, FFS, or other agreed upon payment method between pharmacist and physician or patient.

Medicare *annual wellness visits* (AWV) are a yearly appointment with a provider to create or update a personalized prevention plan. The physician will perform a physical examination and provide any education and diagnostics. The physician and pharmacist will have a clear agreement as to what services will be provided by the pharmacist. The pharmacist's role can include a health risk assessment, medication review, collecting vital signs, social and family history, and conducting various screenings for cognition, hearing, mental health, depression, and fall risk. During an AWV, a pharmacist can provide education on chronic conditions, refer patients at need for further follow-up, and conduct counseling. After collecting this information, the pharmacist and physician will work together to develop a care plan for the patient. Follow-up AWV update the plan from the initial visit and provide further education, and patient referrals may be made as needed. These AWV will need to be billed by the physician under the patient's medical insurance, Medicare provides 100% coverage. In the collaborative care services agreement, the physician and pharmacist will negotiate a reimbursement fee fair to both parties.

For Medicare patients with 2 or more chronic conditions, *chronic care management (CCM)* is another service that can be provided by pharmacists to coordinate care in between provider visits.[27] These services are varied and broad; they can include transitions of care, disease state education, self-care recommendations, or care coordination for social determinants of health. In order to bill for these services through Medicare, a care plan must be developed, and a patient must provide consent for CCM. These services are billed in 20-minute increments per calendar month.[21] Pharmacists participating in CCM are designated as clinical staff under the direction of the billing physician on an incident-to basis.[21] The clinical staff are either employees or working under contract to the billing physician whom Medicare directly pays for CCM services. These CCM services may be modeled as a FFS opportunity as pharmacists and physicians enter into emerging quality and value-based payment models.

Another service that can be provided to Medicare patients is remote physiologic monitoring (RPM) for BP, blood glucose, or weight. Similar to CCM, a patient will need to have a care plan, provide consent, and be completed by a contracted pharmacist under collaborative services agreement. In RPM, the pharmacy or the physician will provide a BP monitor,

blood glucose monitors, or scale to the patient. Initial education on the device is provided by the pharmacist and billed under the physician. These devices must provide real time data to the healthcare provider, and many devices use either Wi-Fi or cellular technology to transmit the data for assessment.

For Medicare patients receiving behavioral health treatment, a pharmacist can provide behavioral health interventions (BHI) that facilitate and coordinate pharmacotherapy, provide counseling, and optimize continuity of care. Again, a care plan must be developed, and consent must be obtained from the patient. The services provided may include assessing treatment adherence, tolerability of medications, and clinic response using validated rating scales (General Anxiety Disorder-7 [GAD-7], Patient Health Questionnaire-9 [PHQ-9]).

As a reminder, collaborative care services may be completed by a contracted pharmacist, but billing for these services must be completed by a physician in most cases. Services may be conducted under direct or general physician supervision depending on service type and location, and based on applicable state law, licensure, and scope of practice. Those interested in learning more about these Medicare services should visit the Medicare Learning Network.[28]

## Anticoagulation Services

Anticoagulation services can be offered in a community pharmacy. CPAs made with local cardiologists or physicians allow pharmacists to make evidence-based dosing adjustments to warfarin by assessing and managing International Normalized Ratio (INR) values, preventing and treating bleeding episodes.[29] In this care model, patients can have their INR reading completed at the pharmacy. The pharmacist would adjust the warfarin dose per protocol, fill and dispense the appropriate dose, and then provide education to the patient. This can also be performed remotely if patients have their own point of care device to check INR. The pharmacist would then communicate with the physician and schedule a follow-up appointment.

Anticoagulation service billing methods may include billing patients directly in a FFS model, incident-to physician billing, or contracts with third-party payers depending upon service model and contract.

## Diabetes Management and Prevention Services

The Diabetes Self-Management Education (DSME) accreditation and the Diabetes Prevention Program (DPP) recognition are available for community pharmacies willing to invest and diversify their current practice to help patients with diabetes achieve behavioral and clinical goals.

DSME services are eligible for patients newly diagnosed with diabetes or newly eligible for Medicare. They can receive 10 h of education over a consecutive 12-month period, 1 h of one-on-one education and 9 h of group classes. After the first year, patients can receive 2 h of group education every 12 months. Pharmacists should refer to the DSME Toolkit created by the Centers for Disease Control and Prevention (CDC) for further guidance.[30,31]

The DPP uses an evidence-based curriculum to conduct 16 weekly group classes over a 6-month timeframe, followed by 6 monthly group classes over the next 6 months.[32] The program coordinator, a trained lifestyle coach, must demonstrate a participant goal of achieving 5–7% of body weight loss and increased physical activity to 150 mins/week in order to gain recognition as an approved DPP site.

Pharmacies in the same chain can be a satellite location from the original accreditation site, and the program coordinator can train technicians, other pharmacists, and healthcare professionals to teach the classes. Pharmacies can bill Medicare Part B and commercial medical insurance for classes conducted in groups, individual, or telehealth classes. Since these services are covered under medical insurance and not under prescription insurance, the pharmacies will need to purchase an additional billing software system. Several software programs are available including OmniSYS®, AthenaHealth®, HabitNu®, and others.

Once the DSME or DPP certificate is obtained from an accrediting body, this is used for billing under Medicare. For each commercial insurer, a credentialing and approval process is required before billing an individual pharmacy.

## Transition of Care (TOC) Programs

Pharmacies can develop contracts with hospitals, assisted living facilities or home health agencies to establish TOC pharmacy services. These services may be billed by using transitional care management (TCM) Current Procedural Terminology (CPT) codes.[33] Contracts for TOC services should allow pharmacists to access the healthcare system's electronic health record system to track and manage patients' therapy. Patients being discharged from the hospital should be contacted by the pharmacist promptly to ensure they have received all ordered discharge prescriptions, perform medication reconciliation, complete a comprehensive medication review, and provide any pertinent patient education. TOC services can be provided in-person at the pharmacy, at the patient's residence, or they may be conducted on the telephone or telehealth platforms as appropriate. Several resources are available for pharmacists interested in implementing a TOC program: BOOST toolkit, Agency for Healthcare Research and Quality (AHRQ) Re-engineered Discharge training program, American Pharmacists Association Transitions of Care Toolkit and ASHP-APhA Medication Management in Care Transitions Best Practices.[34–37]

## ▓ EXAMPLES OF VALUE-BASED PROGRAMS IN THE COMMUNITY PHARMACY

### Diabetes Value-Based Program

In July 2020, a newly formed partnership between Pharmacy Quality Solutions (PQS) and Humana Medicare Advantage was initiated.[38] This outcome-based pilot program is the first of its kind in the United States. As part of the program, Humana Medicare Advantage provides a FFS for pharmacies who conduct A1C testing and provide incentive payments for patients who achieve an A1C less than 9%. This program helps pharmacists manage patient's diabetes, and it is designed to reward pharmacies for optimal diabetes management outcomes evidenced by A1C lowering. This program was launched as an outcomes-based pilot within the EQuIPP® platform, which is used to document these interventions. This innovative model is paving the way for value-based payments to pharmacists in both chain and independent pharmacies.

Blue Cross and Blue Shield of Minnesota, Thrifty White Drug, and Pfizer, leveraged Thrifty White locations and independent pharmacies throughout Minnesota, to help ensure that Blue Cross patients with diabetes received all recommended care, including screenings, immunizations, and support programming.[39] One-on-one engagement with pharmacists included one or more of the following: medication synchronization, to ensure that prescriptions share a common refill date whenever possible; completing or providing referral for hemoglobin A1c (HbA1c) tests; recommending and/or providing immunizations recommended by the Advisory Committee on Immunization Practices (ACIP); educating patients on the importance of using statin medications and collaborating with providers to initiate therapy; screening for tobacco use and initiating tobacco cessation therapy as appropriate. These pharmacist-provided services have shown to improve patient outcomes and reduce healthcare costs.

## TOC Value-Based Program

In April 2020, the Ohio Pharmacists Association joined the UnitedHealthcare Community Plan of Ohio in launching a new program to improve health outcomes.[40] The launch of this program followed the passing of SB 265 that granted "provider status" for Ohio pharmacists. In this program, pharmacists focused efforts on caring for patients transitioning out of the hospital and in the management of chronic diseases such as diabetes and high BP. Pharmacists used their medication expertise to prevent adverse reactions and optimize therapies in collaboration with other healthcare providers to provide a new level

of care to patients. The program tracked 3 specific quality metrics: hospital readmissions, unnecessary prescriptions, and the management of chronic conditions. Pharmacists in the program were able to bill and receive reimbursement for providing patient care services using existing CPT codes for evaluation and management and TCM.[41]

## Asthma Management Value-Based Program

In 2021, Texas pharmacies, both chain and independent, initiated a partnership with a local healthcare network to reduce 30-day readmission rates for asthma exacerbations in high-risk patients.[42] The pharmacists' role was to ensure proper inhaler technique, implement an asthma action plan, assess asthma triggers, identify medication adherence issues, and educate patients, family members, and caregivers. Payment was based on a hybrid model that resulted in both PMPM payment and performance bonus payments for keeping these high-risk patients out of the hospital.

## CPESN Value-Based Programs

CPESN is a clinically integrated group of community pharmacies forging a pathway for value-based contracting in the United States. This network is provider operated, and membership fees are collected. CPESN operates under the Sherman Antitrust Law to aggregate otherwise competitive businesses into one network to provide higher quality care and lower costs to the consumer. The following are examples of the most recent CPESN value-based contracts that are currently available at the time of this publication.[43] These programs have different models for payment including FFS and/or P4P based on outcomes.

### Opioid Management Value-Based Programs

The Idaho Office of Drug Policy partnered with CPESN Idaho pharmacies for a substance abuse grant to prevent drug divergence of excess opioids in the community.[44] The pharmacist's role was to disseminate information to the physicians, dental offices, and surgery centers on appropriate prescribing. Pharmacists educated patients and family members on proper use and disposal. Pharmacists provided patients with drug disposal bags to allow for safe disposal. This program focused on preventing acute opioid use from transitioning to chronic opioid use. Patients were encouraged to pick up a partial quantity of an opioid, versus the whole quantity to prevent drug divergence. The number of opioids not dispensed was tracked to quantify the unlawful channeling of regulated pharmaceuticals from legal sources to the illicit marketplace.

CPESN Oklahoma pharmacies partnered with an employer who is self-insured under the Employee Retirement Income Security Act of 1974 (ERISA). for opioid management services.[45] Pharmacists were responsible for providing education to the patient, checking the prescription drug monitoring program (PDMP) for excess use, verifying indication for opioid use, calculating morphine milligram equivalents (MME), determining appropriate need for naloxone, and documenting the intervention. Pharmacies were paid on a FFS model for the initial consultation and follow-up visits documented in an eCare plan.

### Social Determinants of Health (SDoH) Value-Based Program

In January 2020, North Carolina Medicare Advantage plan partnered with CPESN North Carolina pharmacies for a comprehensive community pharmacy care service set to work with physicians and clinical staff.[46] This care management service set involved SDoH assessments and referral for social services. SDoH encompasses the psychosocial aspect of healthcare including social, behavioral, and environmental issues. This program offers the opportunity for pharmacies to train their technicians and delivery drivers to be community health workers (CHW), whose function includes screening and referring for social services and care coordination. The pharmacies are paid on a PMPM basis.

### Hypertension Value-Based Program

In September 2019, the South Dakota Department of Health contracted with CPESN pharmacies to administer a hypertension program.[47] Pharmacists are working alongside cardiology teams, physicians, and nurses in their area. The program facilitates the delivery of a BP machine to the patient and training on how to use a BP monitor and record their readings. Patients receive a 45-min consult in lifestyle and behavioral modification to effectively manage their BP. Pharmacists create an eCare plan and follow-up with patients on strategies to reduce and maintain goal BP values. The pharmacies are paid an initial per member per initial consultation followed by a P4P fee structure with a built-in payment for a program coordinator.

### Behavioral Health Value-Based Program

A Missouri pharmacy partnered with plans and physicians to create an antipsychotic long-acting injectable (LAI) administration program.[48] Pharmacies leveraged an appointment-based model, or medication synchronization service, for this program. Patients in this program had all chronic medications synced, or filled on the same date, as the LAI. The LAI then becomes the "anchor" medication that all other medications are synced to. Medication synchronization ensures compliance with concurrent medications by filling all prescriptions on the same date to be picked up together. Patients were called 3–7 d prior to their scheduled administration date to confirm the appointment. On the appointment day, patients were screened using the PHQ-9, abnormal involuntary movement scale (AIMS), metabolic screening, and SDoH. The pharmacist assessed efficacy, toxicity of medications, and other barriers to adherence. If no issues were found, the pharmacist administered the LAI and provided patients with the rest of their chronic medications. Patients were referred to the physician for clinical changes, and the CHW for any SDoH concerns. Follow-up calls were completed for first-time users or those for which concerns were identified. This encounter was documented in an eCare plan and provided to prescribers via a communication form. Pharmacists were paid using a FFS model where pharmacists were paid an administration fee and bonus payments if they met certain criteria.

# STEP-BY-STEP COMMUNITY PHARMACY PRACTICE TRANSFORMATION

Many pharmacy owners and managers may not be ready to take the leap into value-based services. This may be due to the investment in time and skills required; but it is mainly because of the change that is needed in both behavior and mindset to develop a sustainable model. Any endeavor to diversify and implement a clinical program should begin with a SWOT (strengths, weakness, opportunities, threats) analysis of the current scenario. Strengths may include the physical pharmacy location and relationships within the community. Weaknesses may include the cost of equipment, personnel, and time required to initiate the project. Opportunities within the community may include gaps in care such as high hospital readmissions for heart failure. Threats may be competing programs in your area, e.g., a DSME program at a hospital 3 miles away. For more information, see Chapter 2, "Entrepreneurship and Intrapreneurship."

Flip the Pharmacy (FtP) is a program supported by the CPESN USA and the Community Pharmacy Foundation to help advance the community pharmacists' role by developing best practices, sample documents, and resources.[49] FtP weaves innovative practices into the daily workflow to improve patient care and workflow efficiencies. This program also helps demonstrate how to document value provided to the patient and patient outcomes in an eCare plan to track outcomes for payments.

Pharmacies employing FtP follow 6 domains to transform workflow practice, including utilizing the appointment-based model, improving patient follow-up and monitoring, engaging non-pharmacist support staff, optimizing technology, establishing work relationships, and developing a business model. The 6 domains are explained below utilizing an example opioid management implementation protocol for pharmacies,[50,51] illustrated in Figure 11-1.

1. Leverage the appointment-based model
   Scalable pharmacy practice transformation requires changes to workflow, care processes, and business modeling in repeatable, consistent, and achievable increments. Implementation of a clinical program should start with medication synchronization, also called medsync. Medsync allows patients to schedule to pick up all of their medications at one time. Monthly calls are made to check in with the patient to verify their medication list 5 d before refills are due; this call is also made to verify the scheduled pick up date. Any issues such as refill requests and inventory are resolved in these 5 d so the patient can pick up all medications at once. This high touch-point with the patient can now be a springboard for providing other clinical services (e.g., counseling on opioid safety and pain management). This process is called the appointment-based model. The pharmacy leverages the medsync pick-up to discuss patient care needs and help patients reach their medical goals. In the case of opioid management, the patient's other chronic medications can be synchronized with the opioid medication as "the anchor drug."

2. Improve patient follow-up and monitoring
   While reviewing an opioid prescription order, prior to pick up, the pharmacist would calculate MME, verify diagnosis code/indication, check the PDMP, and document the encounter in an eCare plan.

   For this example, the pharmacy staff should identify patients that have been prescribed opioids and assess the patient's risk and safety using an assessment tool such as the Risk Index for Overdose or Serious Opioid-Induced Respiratory Depression (RIOSORD) tool.[52] When appropriate, pharmacists should offer naloxone and communicate patient acceptance/refusal to the prescriber. This encounter should be documented in an eCare plan. For an acute opioid prescription, especially post-surgery, follow-up should include counseling the patient on the risks of opioid use.

# Progression 2: Road Map

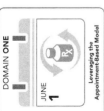

**DOMAIN ONE**

JUNE
1

Leveraging the Appointment-Based Model

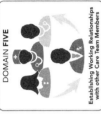

**DOMAIN TWO**

Improving Patient Follow Up and Monitoring

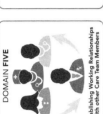

**DOMAIN THREE**

Developing New Roles for Non-Pharmacist Support Staff

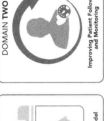

**DOMAIN FOUR**

Optimizing the Utilization of Technology and electronic Care Plans

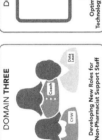

**DOMAIN FIVE**

Establishing Working Relationships with other Care Team Members

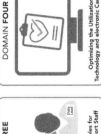

**DOMAIN SIX**

Developing the Business Model and Expressing Value

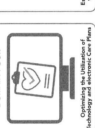

## JUNE
### Appointment-Based Model

- Identify Sync Patients prescribed an opioid
- Calculate MME
- PDMP Check

## JULY
### Improving Patient Follow up and Monitoring

- Continue identifying patients with prescribed opioids
- Assess patient risk and safe use of opioids. Offer naloxone when appropriate
- Send prescriber a note about patient receiving/denying naloxone

## AUGUST
### Non-Pharmacist Support Staff

- Engage technicians with PDMP checks (based on state) & MME Calculation
- Implement pharmacy policy for opioid dispensing and share Opioid Pledge with patients
- Review the roles of staff members and be sure to maximize their roles

## SEPTEMBER
### Optimizing the Utilization of Technology and electronic Care Plans and Establishing Working Relationships with other Care Team Members

- Provide education about acute opioids and safe opioid disposal
- Assess patient's pain control using an assessment
- Enhance prescriber communication
- Review the first 3 Domains and solidify processes

## OCTOBER
### Developing the Business Model and Expressing Value

- Understand your data related to opioids
- Understand the generation of review new opportunities (e.g., grants) based on patient population

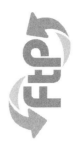

**Figure 11-1.** FtP six transformation domains example.

3. Develop new roles for pharmacist's support staff
   Technicians can identify patients receiving an opioid prescription and flag the prescription, identifying that the patient needs counseling about the pharmacy's opioid pledge.[53] Pharmacies should create and implement a safe opioid dispensing policy/pledge to be shared with patients that highlights the patient's and pharmacists' responsibilities when an opioid is prescribed to a patient, e.g., early dispensing, checking PDMP, and safe drug disposal. This policy would provide guidance regarding patient education and identification of opioid abuse. Technicians can be engaged in the opioid program by completing a state PDMP check, verifying diagnosis code, calculating MME for opioid prescriptions, and starting documentation (in the eCare plan, on the prescription, and in the pharmacy software). At prescription drop off, technicians can be a part of screening for acute prescription opioid use and offering the patient the option to pick up a partial quantity if desired. At prescription pick-up, the technician can educate the patient about the pharmacy opioid dispensing policy while the pharmacist provides specific medication counseling.

4. Optimize the utilization of technology and eCare plans[54]
   Technology can be used to make the pharmacy workflow more efficient. When reviewing prescriptions, technology (such as the PDMP) can be used to easily assess the patient's MME. Other technology can be used to record and track the patient's pain assessment score or the date when an opioid was tapered. The technology used should integrate into the eCare plan platform and the pharmacy management system. Choosing an eCare plan vendor compatible with the pharmacy's dispensing software will enable a smooth workflow, prompting alerts for greater than 50 MME per day, history of naloxone acceptance/denial, history of pledges completed/offered, and any physician instruction for tapering.

5. Establishing work relationships with other team members
   Utilizing the technology features above, the pharmacist can create a spreadsheet that lists all opioids prescriptions, with important information, such as prescribing physician, MME, naloxone accepted/denied, medsync enrollment, and other relevant data. This aggregate data can be used to prepare an infographic for a face-to-face meeting and business proposal with a specific physician, or physicians group. Presenting the infographic, while explaining how pharmacists can impact the MIPS and quality measures of the physician, can be the beginning of a bidirectional referral relationship between the pharmacy and the physician. Sharing eCare plan data and speaking the same care planning language while communicating about mutual patients will be essential for building and retaining sustainable relationships.

6. Developing a business model and expressing value
   One example of a model that can be used is the development of an opioid use disorder (OUD) program. Collaboration with pharmacy and physicians may include the promotion of patient adherence to medications used to treat OUD such as buprenorphine, methadone, or naltrexone. This model could also include naloxone distribution and screening for SDoH issues for referral to case managers.

## ■ ACKNOWLEDGMENTS

The chapter authors would like to acknowledge the following for their expertise in this field and advisement, Troy Trystad, Executive Director CPESN USA, Trista Pfeiffenberger, Director of Operations and Quality CPESN USA, Anne Marie (Sesti) Kondic, PharmD, Executive Director Community Pharmacy Foundation, Ben McNabb, Owner of Love Oak Pharmacy and Lead Luminary of CPESN-Texas.

# CHAPTER APPLICATIONS

1. You are the pharmacy manager of an independent pharmacy located in a small town. Large chain pharmacies are moving in and trying to buy your pharmacy and others in the area. Your pharmacy owner wants to sell the pharmacy due to increasing DIR fees. This change has forced the pharmacy to sell many medications below cost. In the past 6 months, many patients have transferred to others because your pharmacy was not in their insurance's preferred network. Because you are no longer in-network, their prescriptions were no longer covered at your pharmacy. You have recently graduated from pharmacy school and convinced the owner to offer value-based services as an alternative payment model to help the pharmacy stay local and stay in business. The pharmacy owner admits that the pharmacy has a low star rating and he is overwhelmed by the task of improving the pharmacy's star ratings while staying in business. What are some initial steps that the pharmacy can take to improve star ratings and what services can be initiated based on the information provided?

2. After successfully initiating one of the services suggested in Question 1, you have researched the patient demographic of your county. The majority of the patients you serve live in a local retirement community with 60% of the population greater than 65. What other research would be needed to determine the type of additional programs that could be implemented?

3. If your patient population in Question 2 was college-aged patients, how would the value-based programs offered differ?

4. DB is a 57-year-old female who has a family history of diabetes. She is 5′4″ and weighs 175 pounds. DB's most recent A1C = 5.7%. What type of value-based program would you recommend for her?[55,56]

5. Eight years later, DB (from Question 4) has returned to your pharmacy for a point-of-care A1c test with a result of 8.9%. DB's current medication profile includes metformin 1000 mg BID. When inquiring about complications of diabetes she states that she has numbness in her feet. What type of value-based program would you recommend for her based on her insurance benefits?

6. You have spoken to Dr. Healthy, the chief medical officer of the local healthcare system, to set up a contract to start a community pharmacy-based BP monitoring program for their high-risk patients at your pharmacy. The payment will follow an outcomes-based model for bonus payments of $100 per patient if 80% of the referred patients achieve a BP goal < 130/80 mmHg. How will you start implementing this program into the workflow? How will you utilize pharmacists, technicians, and technology?

# REFERENCES

1. Rite Aid announces first closing of asset sale to Walgreens Boots Alliance. Riteaid. Published November 27, 2017. Accessed October 4, 2020. https://www.riteaid.com/corporate/investor-relations/quarterly-results/-/pressreleases/rite-aid-enters-into-an-agreement-with-walgreens-boots-alliance-to-sell-2-186-rite-aid-stores-and-related-assets-for-5-175-billion

2. LaVito A. Walgreens cuts jobs at its US headquarters as drugstore chain slashes costs. *CNBC*. Published October 28, 2019. Accessed October 4, 2020. https://www.cnbc.com/2019/10/28/walgreens-cuts-jobs-at-its-us-headquarters-as-drugstore-cuts-costs.html

3. CMS. National Health Expenditures 2017 Highlights. Published 2017. Accessed October 4, 2020. https://www.cms.gov/research-statistics-data-and-systems/statistics-trends-and-reports/nationalhealthexpenddata/downloads/highlights.pdf

4. Federal Trade Commission. Clinical Integration in Antitrust: Prospects for the Future. Published September 17, 2007. Accessed September 30, 2020. https://www.ftc.gov/sites/default/files/documents/public_statements/clinical-integration-antitrust-prospects-future/070917clinic_0.pdf

5. Federal Trade Commission. Clinical Integration: The Changing Policy Climate and What it Means for Care Coordination. Published April 27, 2009. Accessed January 29, 2021. https://www.ftc.gov/sites/default/files/documents/public_statements/clinical-integration-changing-policy-climate-and-what-it-means-care-coordination/090427ahaclinicalintegration.pdf

6. Adherence. Pharmacy Quality Alliance. Alexandria, VA. Updated March 25, 2021. https://www.pqaalliance.org/adherence-measures

7. EQuIPP. Accessed September 30, 2020. http://www.equipp.org/

8. Terrie YC. Vaccinations: The expanding role of pharmacists. *Pharmacy Times.* 2010;76(1).

9. Weaver KK. Pharmacist-administered immunizations: What does your state allow? *Pharmacy Today.* October 2015:62–63.

10. ITA National Travel & Tourism Office. TI Outreach: Outbound Overview Outbound. Accessed September 30, 2020. https://travel.trade.gov/outreachpages/outbound.general_information.outbound_overview.asp

11. Hamer DH, Connor BA. Travel health knowledge, Attitudes and practices among United States travelers. *J Travel Med.* 2004;11(1):23–26. doi:10.2310/7060.2004.13577

12. Hurley-Kim K, Goad J, Seed S, Hess K. Pharmacy-based travel health services in the United States. *Pharmacy.* 2018;7(1):5–16. doi:10.3390/pharmacy7010005

13. Larrick Chavez-Valdez A. CY 2020 Medication Therapy Management Program Guidance and Submission Instructions. Published April 5, 2019. Accessed September 30, 2020. https://www.cms.gov/Medicare/Prescription-Drug-Coverage/PrescriptionDrugCovContra/Downloads/Memo-Contract-Year-2020-Medication-Therapy-Management-MTM-Program-Submission-v-041019-.pdf

14. Joint Commission of Pharmacy Practitioners. Pharmacists' Patient Care Process. Published May 29, 2014. Accessed October 18, 2020. https://jcpp.net/wp-content/uploads/2016/03/PatientCareProcess-with-supporting-organizations.pdf

15. CY 2021 Medication Therapy Management Program Guidance and Submission Instructions. Published May 22, 2020. Accessed May 14, 2021. https://www.cms.gov/files/document/memo-contract-year-2021-medication-therapy-management-mtm-program-submission-v-052220.pdf

16. Pattah V. MTM and the CMR completion rate: What community pharmacists need to know. *America's Pharmacist.* June 2015:35–36.

17. Pharmacy Quality Alliance. PQA Quality Measures. Updated March 5, 2021. Accessed April 21, 2021. https://www.pqaalliance.org/pqa-measures

18. Pharmacy Quality Alliance. Medication Management Services. Updated March 17, 2021. Accessed May 28, 2021. https://www.pqaalliance.org/medication-management-services

19. Pharmacy Quality Alliance. PQA Measures Overview. Published February 27, 2020. Accessed September 30, 2020. https://www.pqaalliance.org/assets/Measures/PQA_Measures_Overview.pdf

20. Pharmacist eCare Plan Initiative. Accessed April 15, 2021. https://www.ecareplaninitiative.com/

21. Centers for Medicare and Medicaid Services. Chronic Care Management Services. Published July 2019. Accessed October 18, 2020. https://www.cms.gov/outreach-and-education/medicare-learning-network-mln/mlnproducts/downloads/chroniccaremanagement.pdf

22. Billing Guidance for Pharmacists' Professional and Patient Care Services. National Council for Prescription Drug Programs, Inc. Published June 2018. Accessed November 5, 2020. https://www.ncpdp.org/NCPDP/media/pdf/WhitePaper/Billing-Guidance-for-Pharmacists-Professional-and-Patient-Care-Services-White-Paper.pdf?ext=.pdf

23. Pham K. Alternative payment approaches for advancing comprehensive medication management in primary care. *Pharmacy Practice.* 2020 October;18(4).

24. Medicare.gov. Yearly "Wellness" visits. Accessed October 18, 2020. https://www.medicare.gov/coverage/yearly-wellness-visits

25. Centers for Medicare and Medicaid Services. Collaborative Practice Agreements and Pharmacists' Patient Care Services: A Resource for Pharmacists. Published October 2013. Accessed October 18, 2020. https://www.cdc.gov/dhdsp/pubs/docs/translational_tools_pharmacists.pdf

26. Preventive and screening services. Centers for Medicare & Medicaid Services. Accessed November 5, 2020. https://www.medicare.gov/coverage/preventive-screening-services

27. Chronic Care Management. American Pharmacists Association. Washington, DC. https://portal.pharmacist.com/chronic-care-management

28. Centers for Medicare and Medicaid Services. Medicare Learning Network. Accessed April 14, 2021. https://www.cms.gov/Outreach-and-Education/Medicare-Learning-Network-MLN/MLNGenInfo

29. Milam SK. Anticoagulation monitoring: The next community pharmacy value proposition. *Pharm Times.* 2014;1(4).

30. Centers for Disease Control and Prevention. Diabetes Self-Management Education and Support (DSMES) Toolkit. Published March 6, 2018. Accessed August 19, 2020. https://www.cdc.gov/diabetes/dsmes-toolkit/index.html

31. National Diabetes Prevention Program Coverage Toolkit. Published November 26, 2020. Accessed August 19, 2020. https://coveragetoolkit.org/

32. Centers for Disease Control and Prevention. Diabetes Prevention Program. Accessed on August 19, 2020. https://www.cdc.gov/diabetes/prevention/index.html

33. Somma McGivney M, Krahe Dombrowski S. Billing Primer: A Pharmacist's Guide to Outpatient Fee-for-Service Billing. Published August 2019. Accessed October 22, 2020. https://elearning.pharmacist.com/products/5185/aphas-billing-primer

34. Project BOOST Implementation Guide. 2nd ed. Society of Hospital Medicine; 2013. https://www.hospitalmedicine.org/globalassets/professional-development/professional-dev-pdf/boost-guide-second-edition.pdf

35. Jack B, Paasche-Orlow M, Mitchell S, Forsythe S, Martin J, Brach C. Re-Engineered Discharge (RED) Toolkit. Published March 2013. Accessed October 22, 2020. https://www.ahrq.gov/patient-safety/settings/hospital/red/toolkit/index.html

36. American Pharmacists Association. Transitions of Care Toolkit. Accessed October 22, 2020. https://www.pharmacist.com/Practice/Patient-Care-Services/Transitions-of-Care

37. ASHP-APhA Medication Management in Care Transitions Best Practices. Published February 2013. Accessed May 28, 2021. https://www.ashp.org/-/media/assets/pharmacy-practice/resource-centers/quality-improvement/learn-about-quality-improvement-medication-management-care-transitions.ashx

38. Business Wire. Pharmacy Quality Solutions and Humana Partner to Launch New Outcomes-Based Pilot Program. Published June 15, 2020. Accessed October 1, 2020. https://www.businesswire.com/news/home/20200615005020/en/Pharmacy-Quality-Solutions-Humana-Partner-Launch-New

39. Minnesota Pharmacists Successfully Intervene to Close Care Gaps for Patients with Diabetes. Published December 9, 2020. Accessed May 13, 2021. https://mncm.org/minnesota-pharmacists-successfully-intervene-to-close-care-gaps-for-patients-with-diabetes/

40. Ohio Pharmacists Association. Pharmacists tapped by UnitedHealthcare to expand access to care and help improve health outcomes in Ohio. Accessed October 1, 2020. https://www.ohiopharmacists.org/aws/OPA/pt/sd/news_article/293763/_PARENT/layout_interior_details/false

41. Bonner L. Medicaid managed care plans start paying Ohio pharmacists as providers. *Pharmacy Today.* 2020;26(9):34. doi:10.1016/j.ptdy.2020.08.013

42. CPESN Texas. Ben McNabb. Accessed May 13, 2021. https://vimeo.com/showcase/7683386/video/537734831

43. CPESN Payer Success Videos. Accessed May 13, 2021. https://vimeo.com/showcase/cpesn

44. CPESN Idaho. Lorri Shaver. Accessed May 13, 2021. https://vimeo.com/showcase/7683386/video/445900887

45. RxSelect CPESN. Courtney Lundeen. Accessed May 14, 2021. https://vimeo.com/showcase/7683386/video/443245930

46. Mutual CPESN. Patrick Brown shares another payer Program experience. Accessed May 14, 2021. https://vimeo.com/showcase/7683386/video/441511997

47. CPESN South Dakota. Josh Ohrtman. Accessed May 14, 2021. https://vimeo.com/showcase/7683386/video/546493488

48. Levy S. Independents raise the bar. *Drug Store News.* March 2021:80–83.

49. Flip the Pharmacy. Accessed October 4, 2020. https://www.flipthepharmacy.com/

50. Nguyen N, Tucker A. Implementing an Opioid Protocol. Published March 8, 2021. Accessed October 23, 2020. https://vimeo.com/456794508

51. Flip the Pharmacy. What is a Change Package? Accessed October 4, 2020. https://www.flipthepharmacy.com/change-packages

52. Raouf M. Pain Awareness Month: Pharmacist Assessment of Opioid Overdose Risk. Pain Awareness Month: Pharmacists Assessment of Opioid Overdose Risk. Published September 1, 2015. Accessed October 11,

2020. https://www.pharmacytimes.com/contributor/jeffrey-fudin/2015/09/pain-awareness-month-pharmacist-assessment-of-opioid-overdose-risk

53. CPESN Networks. Guidance for Community-Based Pharmacists: Developing a Patient Opioid Pledge. Accessed October 22, 2020. https://162fba55-f60b-49ce-ac53-d43a5ce442ab.usrfiles.com/ugd/162fba_3cacba06e3964c1eb0d93887a806797c.pdf

54. Pharmacist eCare Plan Initiative. Accessed April 15, 2021. https://www.ecareplaninitiative.com/

55. Centers for Disease Control and Prevention. National Diabetes Prevention Program—About the National DPP. Published November 15, 2018. Accessed September 24, 2020. https://www.cdc.gov/diabetes/prevention/about.htm

56. National Institute of Diabetes and Digestive and Kidney Diseases. Diabetes Prevention Program (DPP). Accessed May 30, 2020. https://www.niddk.nih.gov/about-niddk/research-areas/diabetes/diabetes-prevention-program-dpp

# CHAPTER APPLICATION SOLUTIONS

## CHAPTER 1

1. For questions related to patient care services, such as medication administration, you should reach out to the Patient Care Manager or Patient Care Team. The Patient Care Manager's role includes managing patient care services for a geographic area and this would include being familiar will patient care protocols. The Patient Care Team is another option since these members of the team provide patient care services. Since medication administration services are offered by the organizations and are legal in the state, a member of the Patient Care Team should be familiar with the medication administration service, including the protocol. Another option would be to ask the Regional Pharmacy Manager. The Regional Pharmacy Manager manages the business components of the pharmacy and should be familiar with patient care services that are offered at this location. Finally, you could ask the Director of Pharmacy Operations; however unless you have an established relationship with the Director you would want to contact the Director of Pharmacy Operations as a last resort.

2. Examples of currently offered operational services: prescription filling, medication evaluation, patient safety, prescription delivery, inventory management, personnel management. Examples of currently offered patient care services: Routine and travel immunizations, disease state management, medication therapy management, medication administration, and pharmacist prescribing services.

3. Examples of Community-based Pharmacist Practitioner services: execute the JCPP—Pharmacists' Patient Care Process, conduct medication reconciliation during the prescription filling process, evaluate the appropriateness of medications during the prescription filling process, resolve therapy issues (e.g., drug-drug, drug-disease, drug-allergy interactions) through the Drug Utilization Review (DUR) process, identify, and recommend patient care services (e.g., immunizations, MTM services, disease state management services), recommend over-the-counter (OTC), herbal, and natural products, triage and answer patient disease state and medication related questions, refer patients to other healthcare providers (e.g., Emergency Department, Primary Care Provider, Dentist), prescribe medications, collaborate with other healthcare providers to optimize therapies and offer patient care services within the community at health fairs, and so on.

4. Since constructing a drive through window is not an option, an alternative would be to offer medication delivery services. This option is not cost prohibitive since it does not require construction. However, you will need dedicated space to prepare shipping packages, ultimately optimizing patient safety. The pharmacy will need a dedicated location to prepare and ship prescription orders, which may include both prescription and OTC products.

5. In addition to cost, the pharmacy should ensure that they have adequate space to house the automated system. Automated machines can take up a considerable amount of space within the pharmacy.

## CHAPTER 2

1. The scenario at the beginning of the chapter presents two options which are best described as "entrepreneurship" and "intrapreneurship." Both deal

with the concept of "extracting value"—which essentially means finding new ways to provide services or products which customers want to purchase. However, intrapreneurship takes entrepreneurial skills and applies them within an existing organization. It has less inherent risk than entrepreneurship—as almost all risk, especially financial risk, is borne by the pharmacy organization and not by you yourself. However, not all organizations foster, promote, or encourage intrapreneurship—and many which do, still ultimately may not agree with your vision or ideas. Weighing the positives and negatives of both in your specific situation is critical because at face value there really is no advantage of one over the other. It is only when you apply it to a specific case or situation that you begin seeing one emerge as the better choice.

2. When weighing the options of staying with an organization where quality of work life is poor in hopes of helping the organization improve (intrapreneurship) versus striking out on your own and owning your own pharmacy (entrepreneurship), you must carefully think through both scenarios. If you have innovative ideas for the pharmacy and believe that the resources available to your current employer would help ensure success—then perhaps intrapreneurship is right for you. However, those same good ideas may make your own pharmacy more successful—and if they're less resource intensive, then maybe it could offer you a competitive edge over larger competitors. For instance, if your idea is to develop a medication synchronization and packaging service which centrally fills and packs all patient medications at a central location and then distributes to other pharmacies in the organization, then one or two independent pharmacies are not enough to make this idea work (business model failure). Moreover, the buildout of such an idea may exceed the resources (startup and working capital) you have in the first few years of your pharmacy.

3. The idea of a junior partnership is a well-established small business model which exists beyond pharmacy and can be seen across most industries. In short, the junior partnership model provides you time to grow your expertise and financial readiness to own your own pharmacy. Given the scenario at the beginning of the chapter, it can be thought of as an in-between your entrepreneurship and intrapreneurship pathways: a middle road. You do not own the pharmacy, though you may own a small share of it. This means that although your ideas for running the business may be more valued and accepted than by your current chain pharmacy, they still are ultimately up to the current pharmacy owner. There is an increase in autonomy, but you are not yet "your own boss." There is still financial risk, but the majority of that risk is borne by the current senior pharmacy owner (who owns the majority of the shares).

4. Innovation is the development of a new way to provide a process, service, or product to a patient or customer—ideally to improve their overall customer or patient experience. Some individuals may be more innately innovative than others. We often think of these individuals as creative and "out of the box" thinkers. However, even if some of this innovative skillset is genetic, the majority of innovation skills are not due to genes alone. Like most skills (e.g., riding a bike, giving an immunization) it can be refined over time by using best practices—those things that proven innovators do better than others which makes them successful.

5. Innovation can be refined—regardless of how innately innovative you consider yourself. There are five main innovation skills used by today's top innovators which can be performed and improved by anyone, regardless of their innovation start point. These include associating, questioning, observing, experimenting, and networking—and definitions are given within the chapter. For example, by networking with other pharmacy owners at a national pharmacy owner conference, you learn that someone on the other side of the country has developed a new process which has

boosted patient adherence rates by 33%—which is important to you because it means improved insurance company network access and the potential for bonus payments in addition to being good patient care. You may also practice questioning—asking "why" with every customer complaint that comes to you. Why was the prescription late? The pharmacist was busy. Why was the pharmacist busy? The technician was working on an insurance billing problem with another technician. Why were two technicians working on the same problem? There is perhaps inadequate training on insurance billing.

6. A business model is your "best guess" at why patients or customers will give you their money. Although seemingly straightforward, it can be frustratingly challenging to pinpoint. Not only do business leaders mistake the true "why" or "how" their business model works, but customers too are sometimes confused at why they shop at a given business. For example, Walmart is well known for having low prices, but historically terrible customer service. Most likely you or someone you know, if asked, would complain about a recent Wal-Mart customer service experience. However, Wal-Mart continues to be a thriving, successful retail store despite its poor reputation for customer service. How can this be? Well, even though customers will state their need for a high level of customer service, their BEHAVIORS demonstrate that they value low prices over their desire for customer service. Wal-Mart knows this, even if their customers do not, because they have been strategic in thinking through their business model. One way to assist a pharmacist in thinking through their business model in this strategic way is to use a business model canvas—a visual, one-page depiction of how various aspects of the business can come together to form the business model. As opposed to a narrative description of the model, the canvas is meant to allow you to quickly glance at the entire business and how it serves the needs of its customers. In other words,

it is meant to help you see the bigger picture more clearly—a picture that may get lost in the fine print of a business plan.

7. The opening or purchase of a pharmacy is an intimidating prospect. However, more than that, it is one which carries with it significant financial risk for all parties invested in its success—including you, your partners, and investors such as banks. That said, in this scenario you have several things going for you. You have 18 years' experience as a pharmacist, equity in your home which you can borrow against, and a small savings. That said, you also have some things working against you. Although sizable, your savings does not come close to the price of a pharmacy ($500 000-$1 000 000). You're also about half-way through your working career, so a junior partnership may be a less attractive option for you if it's over a longer time horizon like 10 to 15 years and because you already have significant experience built up over the time you have been a pharmacist. So, if you rule out the junior partnership, your options include a home equity loan, a conventional loan, or an SBA-backed loan. Although you have significant equity built up in your home ($150 000), it may be too risky for you and your family to borrow against your house and so you may decide to leave this as an option on the table but leave it as a backup. Given the size of the loan and the relative stability of the independent pharmacy industry, an SBA-backed loan may be the best option at this point in time. The conventional loan option would have been a better choice if your total amount to borrow was less, you had more equity in your house, or more money saved. SBA will serve to partially guarantee the loan on your behalf, thus improving your chances for approval and keeping the overall interest rate affordable. Also, do not forget that both working capital and start-up capital must be accounted for in your financial estimates. You may wish to consider a revolving line of credit, such as a business credit card, for working capital in this scenario.

# CHAPTER 3

1. At minimum, it would be important to include job qualifications and eligibility criteria for the new technician posting. Eligibility criteria includes: an active technician license in good standing and previous work experience with customer-facing responsibilities. Other company-specific requirements, such as minimum age or satisfactory drug screen results should be included as well. Job qualifications include: positive attitude, computer typing skills, and ability to multitask. These characteristics can help prepare candidates for relevant interview questions if selected.

2. $89,500 × 9.8% = $8,771 originally budgeted labor

   $84,000 × 9.8% = $8,232 new budgeted labor

   Difference = $539

   Technician hours: $15 × 25 h = $375

   Clerk hours $10 × 16 h = $160

   25 technician hours will be cut and 10 clerk hours will need to be cut the rest of the week to ensure labor stays at 9.8% of sales.

3. Make time to meet with the pharmacist privately, after their shift has ended. This allows the pharmacist to focus on the conversation at hand and speak in an environment away from other coworkers. Present specific evidence and examples of customer complaints that have been brought to your attention, and ask for the pharmacist's reaction—perhaps there are external factors that are contributing to this trend that you were not aware of. Work to set a mutual plan for improvement and re-training if needed. Be sure to set goals that are measurable, so you can check in periodically to track progress.

4. Speak with Betty first individually. Mention that members of the pharmacy staff have noticed tension between Betty and Carla. Listen to how Betty feels and what emotions she is feeling due to the situation. If Betty is feeling disrespected, ask for specific examples to give to Carla. Speak to Carla individually. State that members of the pharmacy staff have noticed tension between Betty and Carla. Provide examples if necessary and attempt to find the root cause of Carla's behavior. Next, bring Betty and Carla together with another pharmacist or supervisor figure to discuss and resolve their differences. Since you have spoken with them each individually, you should be able to anticipate any conflict that might arise and defuse it quickly and effectively. They need to speak with each other directly and find a solution together with the manager's help.

# CHAPTER 4

Example:

Step 1: Identify 3 to 4 areas of your pharmacy workflow that you would like to improve:

- Provide immunizations on a walk-up basis.
- Decrease wait times.
- Answer phones faster/decrease hold times for customers.
- Check-in orders faster.

Step 2: From this list, select 1 area where improvement is most needed and that will increase your bottom-line profits.

- Provide immunizations on walk-up basis instead of during scheduled clinics

Step 3: For the area of improvement selected, identify:

- WHY: Why are you doing this?
  Customers now want immunizations when it is convenient for them. More and more customers are asking for this and many of your competitors are already doing this. If we can implement this, we will increase the number of immunizations we are giving and this will increase our profits. Doing this will also improve our customer's satisfaction with the services we provide.

- WHAT: What are you promising?

  Customers will now be able to come into our pharmacy anytime we are open and receive immunizations. This service will now be integrated into our regular pharmacy workflow. Because demand can vary we would like to avoid adding extra payroll hours. We also want to maintain our current service standards and do not want to increase prescription wait times.

- HOW: How are you going to deliver?
  - What needs to be done?
    - Non-pharmacist support staff will assist with workflow to the greatest extent possible in order to save the pharmacists' time.
    - Provide immunizations as part of the regular workflow and immunizations will be treated like prescriptions.
    - Time needed to administer immunizations will be incorporated into prescription wait times.
  - How is it done?
    - Streamline workflow and create/update standard operating procedures (SOPs).
    - Organize supplies to improve efficiency:
      - Move consent forms, vaccine information sheets, and other paperwork needed to drop-off/pick-up windows.
      - Organize immunization area so it looks professional, has the supplies needed to administer immunizations.
    - Train all pharmacy staff on new SOPs.
      - Schedule a pharmacy meeting to review and train entire team on this new process.
  - Who does what? _____
    - In-take Technician/Clerk:
      - Assist customers requesting immunizations. Collect customer information and have customers fill out all paperwork needed. Collect payment as needed.
    - Order Entry Technician:
      - Input all information into the pharmacy system. Prepare immunizations for pharmacists. Gather supplies needed. Draw up immunizations.
    - Pharmacist:
      - Review paperwork and administer immunizations.
  - How do they do it?
    - Will be spelled out in new SOPs.

## ▪ CHAPTER 5

1. The pharmacist cannot fill this prescription order because the prescriber is a dentist, and his prescriptive authority is limited to prescription orders that pertain to the practice of dentistry. Before refusing to dispense the medication, the pharmacist should call the dentist to confirm that the medication is for back pain and not dental pain. If the pharmacist learns that the ICD-10 diagnostic code was mistakenly entered, and that the prescription order was issued for dental pain, the pharmacist should follow his or her state's guidelines for changing information on a prescription order for a Schedule II drug before dispensing the medication. Some states may require that the dentist issue a new prescription with the correct information.

2. The pharmacist may dispense the amount of medication that is sufficient to cover the time needed for the physician to issue a written prescription order (a 2- or 3-day supply in this scenario). This oral authorization for a Schedule II drug is legal because it meets the definition of an emergency: (1) the immediate administration of the controlled substance is necessary for the proper treatment of the patient, (2) no appropriate alternative treatment is available, and (3) it is not reasonably possible for the prescribing physician to provide a written prescription to the pharmacist before dispensing. A pharmacist may accept the oral authorization of a prescribing individual practitioner for a schedule II drug, provided that: (1) the quantity prescribed and dispensed is limited to the amount adequate to treat the patient during

the emergency period, (2) the prescription is immediately reduced to writing by the pharmacist and contains all required information except for the signature of the prescribing individual practitioner, and (3) the pharmacist makes a reasonable effort to determine that the oral authorization came from a registered individual practitioner. Within 7 days after authorizing an emergency oral prescription, the prescribing individual practitioner must provide a written prescription that includes the date of the oral order to the dispensing pharmacist with the notation: "Authorization for Emergency Dispensing." Emergency oral prescription orders for schedule II drugs should be a rare occurrence, particularly now with the mandates for using e-prescriptions for controlled substances.

3. Individuals have a right to access their PHI that is part of the designated record set, which includes billing and payment records. The covered entity, here the pharmacy, must provide access within 30 calendar days, but responding to the request as soon as possible is encouraged. Finally, the covered entity is allowed to impose a reasonable, cost-based fee for the request such as for labor, supplies, and postage that are required to provide the information to the patient in the form and format the patient requested. While the law does permit these fees, this information should be provided for free, especially for patients with financial hardship.

4. HIPAA specifically permits a covered entity to disclose PHI to a health oversight agency, such as a Board of Pharmacy, to conduct activities that the agency is specifically authorized by law to conduct. These activities can be civil, administration, or criminal in nature. Thus, so long as the Board of Pharmacy in the state the pharmacy is located in is specifically authorized to inspect pharmacy practice sites and conduct investigations for possible illegal activity, then pharmacist disclosure of the prescriptions would be permitted.

5. No, you should not sign the agreement. Stark Law is a strict liability law that makes it unlawful for a physician to financially gain from a referral for designated health services. Being the only store in town, it is likely that you would bill Medicare for designated health services, like certain types of medical equipment. Moreover, because the physician has a vested interest in the volume of medical equipment sales, they would benefit directly from any referrals sent to the store. Paying the physician a percentage of the profits would be a violation of Stark law's strict liability and you could personally face exclusion from participation in Medicare and civil money penalties.

6. The manager's plan likely violates the Anti-Kickback Statute (AKS). The AKS prevents an individual from knowingly soliciting or offering remuneration in exchange for a good or service that will be paid in full or part by federal healthcare programs. Here, by advertising the pharmacy is waiving copays in the rewards club, the pharmacy is providing remuneration (the value of a waived copay) in exchange for billing a prescription that may be reimbursed by a federal healthcare program. While there is a safe harbor for waiving copays due to patient financial need, waivers that are blanket, routine, and advertised are not allowed by the statute's safe harbors.

## ■ CHAPTER 6

1. Some example questions for the current Pharmacist-in-Charge (PIC) include:

   - How is the inventory in the pharmacy currently organized?

   - What does the inventory ordering process look like?

   - What tools are in place to help manage and regulate the pharmacy inventory?

   - What preparation is recommended and needed to take inventory?

- When should the change in PIC inventory be scheduled?

Becoming a brand new PIC can be overwhelming, so jotting down questions to ask will help guide the transition. Also, know that you are not going to remember everything to ask; definitely use this chapter as a guide. In the authors' experience, it has been beneficial to ask for the outgoing PIC's contact information. More than likely, they will share their information with you without hesitation because they understand that you will have questions later and can serve as a valuable resource.

2. In the authors' experience, using the *ROP/PAR* method of ordering from a perpetual inventory setup is the most effective method of purchasing inventory. The process is front end loaded with the setup of the perpetual count but makes the daily ordering process much more precise with less time and labor involved. They have used all 4 of these methods in various practice settings over the years. The other 3 methods have more obstacles to overcome and a lot less fine control over the on-hand drugs available for dispensing in a normal community pharmacy setting. There certainly are pharmacy settings where each of these methods are more appropriate than others. For example, if you are running a small pharmacy with a limited formulary and predictable prescription volume, the *order-by-use* method may be more appropriate for you. If you are running a specialty pharmacy with extremely high cost drugs that do not require acute dispensing, the *just-in-time* ordering method may be your best bet. The key is to understand your pharmacy's dispensing model and choose the appropriate method that allows the most economical and efficient inventory management method for your situation.

3. There are two pertinent pieces of the DSCSA that community pharmacies need to understand and apply. First, when purchasing (or wholesaling) inventory, you must capture (or provide) and record the three pieces of transactional data

discussed above, the transactional information, the transactional history and the transactional statement. If you buy from a wholesaler or manufacturer, they will be required to provide this information to you but it is your responsibility to make sure they do. Each of these must be maintained in your pharmacy for six years after receipt for possible inspection. Second, each prescription sold to a patient in your pharmacy must have the lot number and expiration date for every unit that is being dispensed. If you dispense 30 tablets from 3 different manufacturer bottles, this information must be documented for both bottles and maintained for a period of 6 years. Most pharmacies work with a pharmacy software vendor that will capture all of this data and store it as part of their normal workflow. That is the simplest way to approach your requirements. If you choose to do this manually, you must develop a very strict protocol of how you deal with purchases and sales to make sure that you maintain all the required documentation on every transaction. Ask your pharmacy software vendor to handle this for you.

4. Before moving into the new pharmacy as PIC, the authors would want to ensure that all security requirements are met (e.g., the alarm system is activated and the locks on the doors, safe and/or vaults are validated). They would also examine the lighting to ensure that it is well visible, make sure that the pharmacy ventilation is appropriate, and monitor the temperature for a short period to see if United States Pharmacopeia (USP) temperature definitions of the pharmacy are maintained. Next, they would evaluate the pharmacy structure and identify the most efficient workflow process. This will help determine how to organize drugs throughout the pharmacy. Drug organization is dependent on pharmacy employee work stations and their ease of accessibility. In the authors' experience, it is more productive to organize drugs in the pharmacy alphabetically by name regardless if it's brand or generic. This is beneficial for rookie staff when trying to locate a drug in production

since they may not be familiar with brand or generics. You definitely want to ensure that workflow is as efficient as possible and that pharmacy production staff are not spending the majority of their time walking around the pharmacy to retrieve drugs. After that, you would need to make sure that you have enough space in a safe or a vault for medications that need to be locked up and secured. Lastly, when organizing drugs in the new pharmacy, ensure there is reasonable space between drugs on the shelf to prevent clutter and to make product amounts visible to help ordering and inventory management.

5. An example inventory checklist would include the following items listed below.

Two weeks before inventory:

❏ Identifying efficient technicians and preparing a team to help conduct the inventory.
❏ Organizing prescription shelves and cleaning the pharmacy.

One week before inventory:

❏ Separating expired medications (while separating controlled substances from legend drugs)
❏ Selecting the day and time inventory will be taken and who will be present.
❏ Determine the best form of inventory record to be used when taking inventory (the authors prefer a written inventory record from the start in order to make notes).
❏ Review any specific state or company requirements regarding inventory procedures.

Day of Inventory:

❏ The inventory team conducts an exact count of all controlled substances listed in Schedule II.
❏ The inventory team conducts an estimated count or measure of all controlled substances listed in Schedules III, IV, and V unless the container holds more than 1000 tablets or capsules, in which case, an exact count of the contents must be made.

❏ Inventory of Schedule II controlled substances is listed separately from the inventory of Schedules III, IV, and V controlled substances.
❏ Perpetual inventory of respective drugs required to be inventoried shall be reconciled on the date of inventory.

After inventory:

❏ Finalize record of inventory, notarize if required, and keep inventory records in pharmacy separate from other records for two years (unless stricter requirements required by state).

# ■ CHAPTER 7

1. Discuss potential options for wearables that measure blood pressure and heart rate like an Omron° monitor and the pros and cons of the different types of devices. Offer to help them evaluate the data the wearable device would collect whenever the patient picks up their refills in the future.

2. Your pharmacy uses a medication synchronization program through its prescription software suite. This allows staff to sync up the patient's medications so they only have to come to the pharmacy once a month to pick up all of their medications. You offer and explain a medication synchronization program to Shirley and tell her you will look at her profile and get everything set up so she only has to run this errand once a month.

3. Examples:
   a. Auto refill.
   b. Med sync.
   c. Text and phone notifications for refills and pickup notifications.
   d. Some or all of the above can be used concurrently.

4. If your pharmacy has the CSOS cloud, the order could be submitted by the pharmacy manager on their smartphone or another registered device without being on-site.

5. The patient should not still be taking the ibuprofen due to the acute use several months ago, but confirm this information while counseling.

# ■ CHAPTER 8

1. At a minimum, the pharmacist would expect to see a balance sheet and an income statement. The balance sheet presents a picture of the pharmacy's financial position at a point in time while the income statement presents the results of operations over a period of time. The two statements are directly linked through the Owner's Equity account which is increased by net income or decreased by net loss.

2. Remodeling a pharmacy is a necessary cost of doing business as it can increase pharmacy operational efficiency by optimizing workflow, and improve a patient's experience which can lead to increased traffic and sales. If the pharmacy has cash reserves for improvements to the store, then one would expect that the current asset "cash" would decrease while the non-current asset "leasehold improvements" (if rented) or "building improvements" (if owned) would increase correspondingly. However, if a loan was required, cash would remain unaffected, but the liability "loans payable" would increase. Note that in neither example is equity impacted. You are either exchanging one asset for another of equal value (cash for a fixed asset) or increasing both assets and liabilities in an equal amount. However, over time one would expect an overall positive impact on the business which may be seen on the income statement through increased profitability and on the balance sheet through increased owner's equity.

3. Your current period purchases were $1 550 000. The formula we learned [Cost of Goods Sold (COGS) = Beginning Inventory (BI) + Purchases (P) − Ending Inventory (EI)] can be rearranged as [P = EI + COGS − BI]. So purchases equal $200 000 + $1 600 000 − $250 000, or $1 550 000. Conceptually, it is important to note that inventory has fallen by $50 000, which means that your sales were composed of your current period purchases (in this example $1 550 000) as well as $50 000 from your opening inventory. You can see here the importance of understanding and managing inventory levels and their relationship to sales in a pharmacy's operations. If sales are greater than purchases over a period, inventory will decrease; if sales are less than purchases, inventory will increase.

4. When dispensing medications in workflow you will often see the cost of the medication and the medication reimbursement (with or without dispensing fee). It would seem that simply subtracting one number from the other would give you an estimate of the pharmacy's profitability. In fact, it is more likely to give you an estimate only of "gross profit." Although useful as a benchmarking tool, it is not an accurate estimate of the overall financial health of a pharmacy. Only after taking into account all expenses that the pharmacy incurs over the year, are you left with the "net income." Net income is always a smaller number than gross profit, and often just a single digit fraction of it (e.g., just 2.5% of total sales in our sample income statement shown in Figure 8-2).

5. The pharmacy's current ratio is [$230 000/$125 000] or 1.84:1. As a rule of thumb, a current ratio of 2:1 or greater is desired. A lesser ratio such as this could be a warning that the pharmacy has over extended its credit or is having difficulty meeting its vendor obligations. The pharmacy's quick ratio is [$50 000 (cash and accounts receivable)/$125 000] or 0.4:1. In general, the quick ratio should be no less than 1:1 indicating the pharmacy has the liquidity to pay its near-term debts. In this example you can see the pharmacy has far fewer liquid assets than obligations and may need to extend supplier payment terms or obtain an infusion of capital. The pharmacy's gross profit margin is [$400 000/$2 000 000] or 20%. While this may seem to be a low number, it is in line with the industry average. Since bottom line profitability flows out of this number, it is important to understand the pharmacy's margins, both overall and product-by-product, increasing sales price and reducing the acquisition cost wherever possible.

6. The planning exercise was attempting to assess risk, perhaps as a component of an overall ERM strategy. As there are many variables which affect a pharmacy's economic success, it is best to eliminate all items which are not within your control so that you may better understand how well the pharmacy is performing based on things that are within your control. The EBITDA metric allows you to do just that—by eliminating extraneous variables which may make it more difficult to understand overall risk and pharmacy performance.

## ■ CHAPTER 9

1. A, B, and C
   a. BSQ01 is the deductible phase which could explain the higher copay.
   b. BSQ02 which is the initial coverage phase could also have coinsurance meaning the patient might have to pay a percentage of the cost, in this case 25%.
   c. BSQ03 is the "donut hole" where the cost of the medication could be higher as well.

2. D. $99.50
   Coinsurance means you pay 25% of the drug cost. So 25% of $398.00 equals $99.50.

3. Yes, the amounts match so the pharmacy was paid correctly according to the contract rate.
   Invokana is a brand medication, so the brand reimbursement formula will apply.

$$AWP = (\$22 \text{ per tablet}) \times 30 = \$660$$

Brand contract
$$\begin{aligned} \text{reimbursement} &= AWP - 18\% + \$0.50 \\ &= \$660 - (\$660 \times 0.18) \\ &\quad + \$0.50 \\ &= \$660 - \$118.80 + \$0.50 \\ &= \$541.70 \checkmark \end{aligned}$$

Actual reimbursement $80 (copay) + $461.70 (Amount paid by Plan) = $541.70 ✔

4. A. What would the pharmacy need to know to be able to develop an action plan to address patient adherence? The pharmacy would need to understand their baseline adherence for patients on this particular plan. First, the pharmacy would identify patients taking a statin over the last year. Then for each patient, the pharmacy would calculate the proportion of days covered. Patients with a PDC of greater or equal to 80% are considered adherent. After the pharmacy would calculate the performance/adherence rate by dividing the number of adherent patients by the total eligible population.

Example: A pharmacy has 22 patients who were on a statin this year for patients of LocalHealthcare—a regional health plan in the area.

Of those 22 patients, 18 had a PDC ≥ 80%, while 4 patients had a PDC score below 80%.

The percent of adherent patients is: 18 ÷ 22 = 81.8%

If the pharmacy maintained the current 81.8% for the upcoming plan year, the DIR fee would be 4% of AWP for each claim under the contract. However, one fewer adherent patient (17 out of 22; 77%) would result in a 7% DIR per prescription. Two additional adherent patients (20 out of 22) would produce a performance score of 90.9% which would result in no DIR being owed to the plan.

B. What action(s) might the pharmacy want to take to improve patient adherence? Once the eligible patients have been identified and a baseline has been established, the pharmacy could take a number of steps to improve patient adherence. For instance, most Medicare plans allow pharmacies to dispense up to a 90 days supply for each claim. Higher days supply can reduce nonadherence. Other examples of tools used by pharmacies to improve adherence are automated refill reminders, medication synchronization and special packaging (e.g., unit dose pouches, talking bottle caps).

# CHAPTER 10

1. Structural elements of care quality at a pharmacy which relate to diabetes care include credentials, such as the Certified Diabetes Educator certification, as well as tangible elements such as glucose meters, A1c point-of-care tests, and clinical management software. If your pharmacy environment lacks any of these elements, adding them allows for expanded care processes related to diabetes care which could improve outcomes.

2. For the 2021 contract year, quality measures include medication adherence for renin-angiotensin system antagonists, statins, and diabetes medications; CMR completion rate; statin use in persons with diabetes; drug plan quality improvement; and 8 measures related to member experience and pricing accuracy. When comparing this list of measures to Table 10-2, the measures included in Table 10-2 are all clinically related. Pharmacists can impact all of these measures, but the hardest to impact may be statin use in persons with diabetes since this requires a new prescription to be written. The drug plan quality improvement measure could be considered impactable by pharmacists since many of the measures which a pharmacist can impact are included in the measure.

3. A good first step is regular monitoring of the EQuIPP platform if this isn't already happening and identify a quality champion who will be in charge of monitoring and leading quality improvement initiatives. Ultimately, working toward a culture which seeks to continuously improve quality will be essential for success, but this can't happen during a rotation experience. Similarly, implementing a service which targets outliers may not be feasible during a rotation, but developing a plan for a service which engages the quality champion in identifying outliers and delivering a targeted intervention could be achievable.

4. There are several different ways that your community pharmacy can work to improve quality measures related to statin use in persons with diabetes (Table 10-3). The first step would be to identify a champion in your pharmacy to lead the pharmacy's quality initiatives and monitor quality. This could be a pharmacist, technician, or other staff members. While a study could lead this effort, the champion would ideally be someone that would be consistent at the pharmacy instead of only there for a rotation. Using the EQuIPP platform or another vendor, the quality champion should run reports regularly to identify patients who are negatively affecting quality scores. The champion can work with pharmacists, technicians, students, and other pharmacy staff to target outreach to these patients. As it was mentioned previously, the quality measure for statin use in persons with diabetes requires a new prescription to be written so developing collaborations with prescribers is important.

5. Community pharmacies have implemented several different solutions to help patients improve their medication adherence when they have transportation issues. One of the most common solutions is medication synchronization. This allows for all of the patient's medication fills to be aligned to the same day of the month. That way the patient only has to find transportation to the pharmacy once a month instead of several times a month. Patients with transportation issues may also benefit from 90-day medication fills. If 90-day medication fills were combined with medication synchronization, the patient would only need to find transportation to the pharmacy every three months. Lastly, some community pharmacies have implemented medication delivery to patients who are unable to make it to the pharmacy to pick up their medications.

# CHAPTER 11

1. To initially increase star ratings at his store the pharmacist can:
   (a) Implement a medication synchronization program

(b) Help increase refill rates by printing a report of medications due to be refilled in the next week. Pharmacy staff can work to call those patients to initiate refills and address any potential adherence issues.

(c) Incorporate MTM into the workflow. Patients that have an active TIP should have their prescription either electronically or manually "flagged" to alert the pharmacy team of additional counseling opportunities. Technicians can help by documenting the outcome of the encounter or they can help schedule CMRs.

(d) Log on to the EQuIPP platform and target the outlier patients who are non-adherent and causing a lower score at the pharmacy.

(e) Implement a compliance packing program. This program can be marketed to patients and caregivers.

(f) Market an MTM program outside of OutcomesMTM® in a cash pay model.

2. The pharmacy team should determine what other disease states are prevalent in their patient population. The team would also want to research prescription usage and type of insurance coverage for the patient population to gauge the type(s) of chronic care management program(s) needed. Also, it is essential to obtain the star ratings and quality measures of the surrounding physicians and hospitals. Based on this information, the newly implemented program should target high-risk patients that are negatively impacting quality metrics for the surrounding facilities and physicians in your area. Remember, that low star ratings mean reduced bonus payments to the physicians. Using this strategy will allow for a quadruple win for the patient, pharmacy, physician and the insurance. A fall prevention program set in a community with high fracture risk is an example of a program that fits the community needs. The pharmacy can work with local physician offices to develop a services agreement that would allow pharmacists to screen seniors for high-risk medications, anticholinergic use, poor cognition, and social determinants of health.

3. This younger age group fits in the bottom 90% of the population that benefits most from convenience care programs (e.g., preventative health and travel health vaccination clinics). The pharmacy can approach self-insured or ERISA companies to offer a DPP program, smoking cessation program, and weight loss program to prevent future healthcare spending.

4. DB has several risk factors for diabetes including being overweight, and family history of diabetes. DB's A1C = 5.7%, she is prediabetic and should be referred to a DPP program at her local pharmacy. DPP programs have been shown to decrease the risk of developing type 2 diabetes by 58% in all age groups and 71% in those over 60 years compared to 31% in those using metformin only.

5. DB has an A1c greater than 6.5% and has complications of diabetes. Because of her diagnosis of diabetes, she should be referred to a diabetes self-management and education program at her local pharmacy. Since DB is now 65, you can assume that she has Medicare coverage. Medicare will allow for DB to receive 10 h of diabetes education.

6. The pharmacist should use the pharmacy's software to run a report to identify patients with hypertension who are managed by the local healthcare system. The pharmacy should approach the healthcare system regarding an adherence monitoring program, for example, medication synchronization. Leveraging the appointment-based model, patients taking hypertension medications and enrolled in medication synchronization should be flagged for counseling on pick up. After addressing issues of adherence, pharmacists can then counsel patients on non-pharmacological interventions for BP lowering. Pharmacists can teach patients how to use their blood pressure monitor, provide education on goal BP values, and supply patients with a BP log.

(a) To improve patient follow-up and monitoring at the next MedSync appointment, pharmacists can assess the patient's BP readings and technique for taking BP. Pharmacists can provide evidence-based recommendations on medication optimization to the physician and document care in an eCare plan.

(b) The pharmacist should develop new roles for support staff. In some states, pharmacy technicians can complete blood pressure readings when patients arrive at the pharmacy. The American Heart Association has an online course, "Achieving Accuracy: BP Measurement," in which healthcare providers can learn how to obtain blood pressure readings. Delivery drivers can also be trained to become a community health worker (CHW) to complete SDoH assessments with patients to identify other social factors that may affect adherence to medications.

(c) The pharmacy team should optimize technology and eCare plans. When a blood pressure is taken by the pharmacy, it should be documented in an eCare plan. The pharmacist should also document the patient's goal BP, education provided, an assessment of the current therapy, plan and follow up.

(d) Prescriber communication is essential to the sustainability of this type of value-based program. Care coordination notes and recommendations within the eCare plan should be sent to the prescribing physician.

(e) Quarterly, pharmacists should share data with prescribers to express the value of the service provided. This document should list the number of patients in the blood pressure monitoring program, the number of these patients enrolled in medication synchronization, the number of patients at goal blood pressure and those that are still uncontrolled. Once this relationship is developed, a bi-directional referral process can be established. A business model can be created where the pharmacy creates a pre-filled prescription pad with clinical services so the physicians can simply check a box for the services that the pharmacy would provide for the patient.

# INDEX

Page numbers followed by "*t*" denote tabular material and those followed by "*f*" denote figures.